Your Horse's Health

Your Horse's Health

A Handbook for Owners and Trainers

Bonnie V. G. Beaver, B.S., D.V.M., M.S.

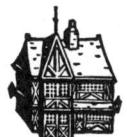

South Brunswick and New York: A. S. Barnes and Company
London: Thomas Yoseloff Ltd

© 1980 by A. S. Barnes and Co., Inc.

A. S. Barnes and Co., Inc.
Cranbury, New Jersey 08512

Thomas Yoseloff Ltd
Magdalen House
136-148 Tooley Street
London SE1 2TT, England

Library of Congress Cataloging in Publication Data
Beaver, Bonnie V G 1944-
   Your horse's health.

   Includes index.
   1. Horses—Physiology. 2. Horses—Diseases.
I. Title.
SF951.B4 636.1'08'9 78-75297
ISBN 0-498-02338-9

PRINTED IN THE UNITED STATES OF AMERICA

To Mom
For immeasurable help and inspiration

Contents

   List of Illustrations

   Preface

1 Equine Shock Absorbers (The Thoracic Limb)   15
2 "P" Is for Push and Pelvic Limb (The Pelvic Limb)   32
3 A Column of Support (The Vertebral Column)   44
4 The Anatomy of a Sigh (The Respiratory System)   47
5 A Ticker at Work (The Circulatory System)   50
6 Eat, Drink, and Be Sick (The Digestive System)   53
7 A Waste Disposal Plant (The Urinary System)   60
8 Foals Don't Come from Eggs (The Genital System)   65
9 Nature's Telephone System (The Nervous System)   81

   Index   85

List of Illustrations

FIGURE 1. Bones of the Thoracic Limb	16
FIGURE 2. Distal Thoracic Limb	18
FIGURE 3. The Hoof	20
FIGURE 4. Cross Section of the Hoof	21
FIGURE 5. Bone Length Affects Muscle Length	22
FIGURE 6. Angulation of the Scapula	23
FIGURE 7. The Foot as a Lever	24
FIGURE 8. Front View of the Thoracic Limbs	26
FIGURE 9. Top View of a Horse	27
FIGURE 10. Foot with Laminitis	27
FIGURE 11. Bones of the Pelvic Limb	33
FIGURE 12. Human Hip Joint	34
FIGURE 13. Horse Hip Joint	35
FIGURE 14. Stifle Joint, Front View	36
FIGURE 15. Types of Surface Contact	37
FIGURE 16. Stifle Joint, Side View	38
FIGURE 17. Angulation of the Pelvic Limb	40
FIGURE 18. Normal and Abnormal Hocks	42
FIGURE 19. Vertebral Column	45
FIGURE 20. A "Typical" Vertebra	46
FIGURE 21. The Diaphragm	49
FIGURE 22. The Kidney	61
FIGURE 23. A Nephron	62
FIGURE 24. Female Reproductive Tract, Top View	66
FIGURE 25. Female Reproductive Tract, Side View	67
FIGURE 26. Male Reproductive Tract, Side View	72
FIGURE 27. Cross Section of a Horse Penis	73
FIGURE 28. Penis and Prepuce	74
FIGURE 29. Fetal Circulation	78
FIGURE 30. The Brain	82

Preface

"Beauty is only skin deep, but ugliness goes plumb to the bone." The shiny coat of the halter-class winner is much more than a reflection of the external products put on it. It indicates the animal's health, including the well-being of all organs. But it takes more than this shiny coat to make a horse a winner. It takes sound well-built legs. *Your Horse's Health* was written with these things in mind, from a veterinarian, educator, and horse enthusiast for the individual who wants to learn more about a horse's inner beauty.

B. V. G. Beaver
Bryan, Texas

Your Horse's Health

1
Equine Shock Absorbers (The Thoracic Limb)

The front leg of the horse receives more physical abuse than any other part of the body, because of its closeness to the animal's center of gravity. Whether landing from a jump or striding in a gallop, all the weight from the animal's body is at some time carried on one slender limb. Its importance therefore cannot be overemphasized.

The bones of the horse actually form the framework onto which the rest of the animal is built, and it should go without saying that good bone structure is essential for a good sound limb.

Starting at the top of the thoracic limb, the area of the shoulder contains a triangularly shaped bone called the *scapula* ("shoulder blade"). The inside of the scapula is generally smooth, but the outside has a tall ridge running down it called the spine. In the normal horse, muscles fill in the area on either side of the spine so that the projection can hardly be felt. Many of you may remember old draft horses who had a shriveling up of the muscles in the shoulder region, a condition called sweeney. In these individuals the spine of the scapula was all too obvious.

The second bone from the top is called the *humerus* located in an area called the *arm*. The top of the humerus has a surface that is convex to fit into the concave, or hollowed out, area at the bottom of the shoulder blade. This area of junction between the scapula and humerus is called the *shoulder joint*, and is located near the *point of the*

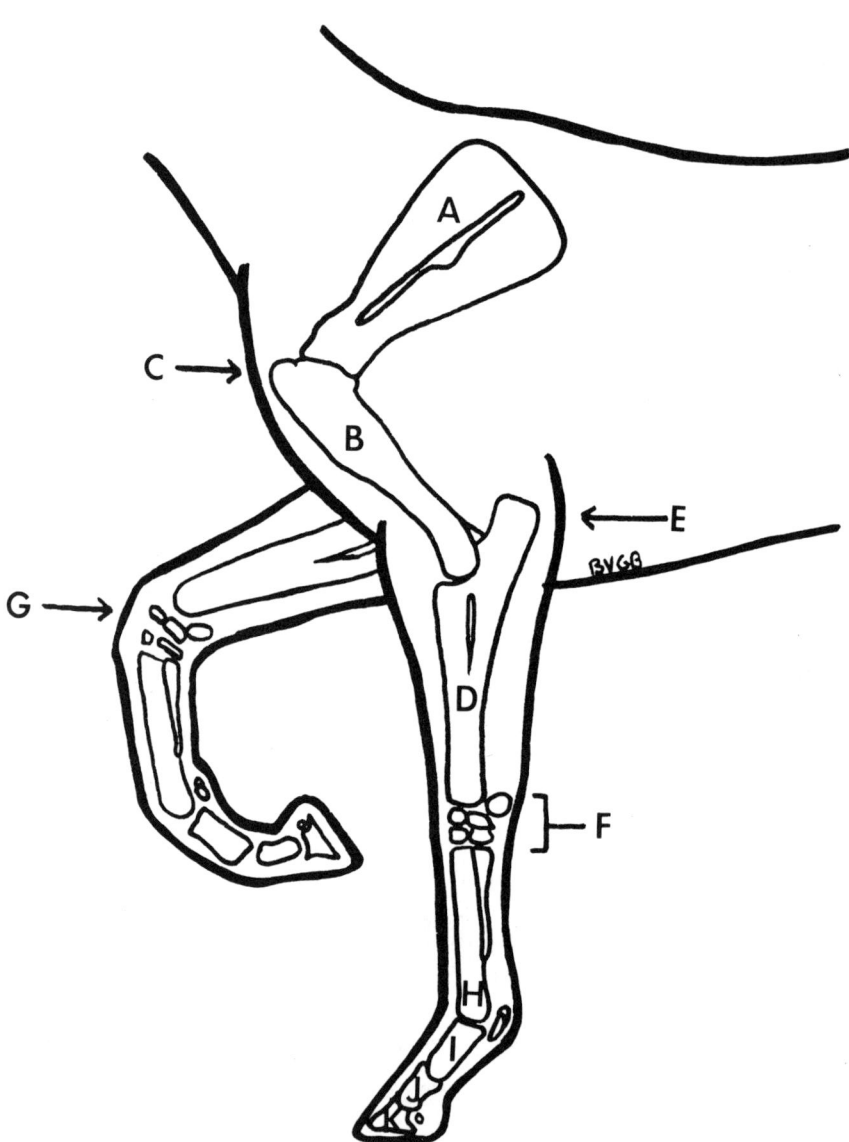

FIGURE 1. **Bones of the Thoracic Limb:** A–Scapula; B–Humerus; C–Point of the Shoulder; D–Radius and Ulna; E–Point of the Elbow; F–Carpus; G–Joints of the Carpus; H–Metacarpal Bone; I–Proximal Phalanx; J–Middle Phalanx; K–Distal Phalanx.

shoulder. The humerus itself is shaped much like a Milk Bone, dog biscuit, with a large part on each end and a thinner shaft in the middle. The bottom is smooth and rounded like a cylinder lying on its side, with the ends pointing sideways. It is this surface that forms half of the *elbow joint*.

The *radius* and *ulna* are fused in the horse to provide more strength. In the front of this bone, about four inches from its top, is a deep notch into which the bottom of the humerus fits—thus the complete elbow joint. The point of the elbow is actually the top of the ulna and not the elbow joint, and it represents the area where a large important muscle attaches. The *forearm*, the area between the point of the elbow and the knee, (the knee of the horse corresponds to the human wrist), is the area where all the muscles that work the lower leg begin.

The bones of the *carpus* ("knee") are located just below the radius and ulna. Racehorses often get fractures or chips of these bones, and it is therefore important to look at this area closer. The horse usually has eight carpal bones arranged neatly into two rows of four bones each, as does the human wrist. In the top row, one bone projects backward. Several muscles attach at this point and other important structures pass through the groove formed just to the inside of this carpal bone.

In the knee, the horse actually has three joints: one between the radius–ulna and the top row of carpal bones; one between the two rows of carpal bones; one between the bottom row of carpal bones and the next bone down, the cannon bone. Only the top two of these joints actually move, the bottom one moving only slightly. If you look at a picture of a parade or three-gaited horse you will notice two bends at the knee, one for each movable joint at the carpus.

The large bone below the knee is called the *third metacarpal* ("cannon") bone, and to each side of it is located a smaller *splint* bone. The cannon bone would be similiar to the bone from the wrist to the middle finger in the human palm. The splint bones are also metacarpal bones, but they are all that is left of the second and fourth toes of earlier ancestors.

The *fetlock joint* is the junction between the cannon bone and the *proximal* ("top") *phalanx* ("long pastern bone"). At the back of the fetlock are two bones sitting side by side, called the *proximal sesamoid bones*. These sometimes fracture in racehorses.

Below the long pastern bone is the *middle phalanx* ("short pastern bone") with the joint between them logically called the *pastern joint*. This bone touches the *distal phalanx* ("coffin bone," "toe bone") at the

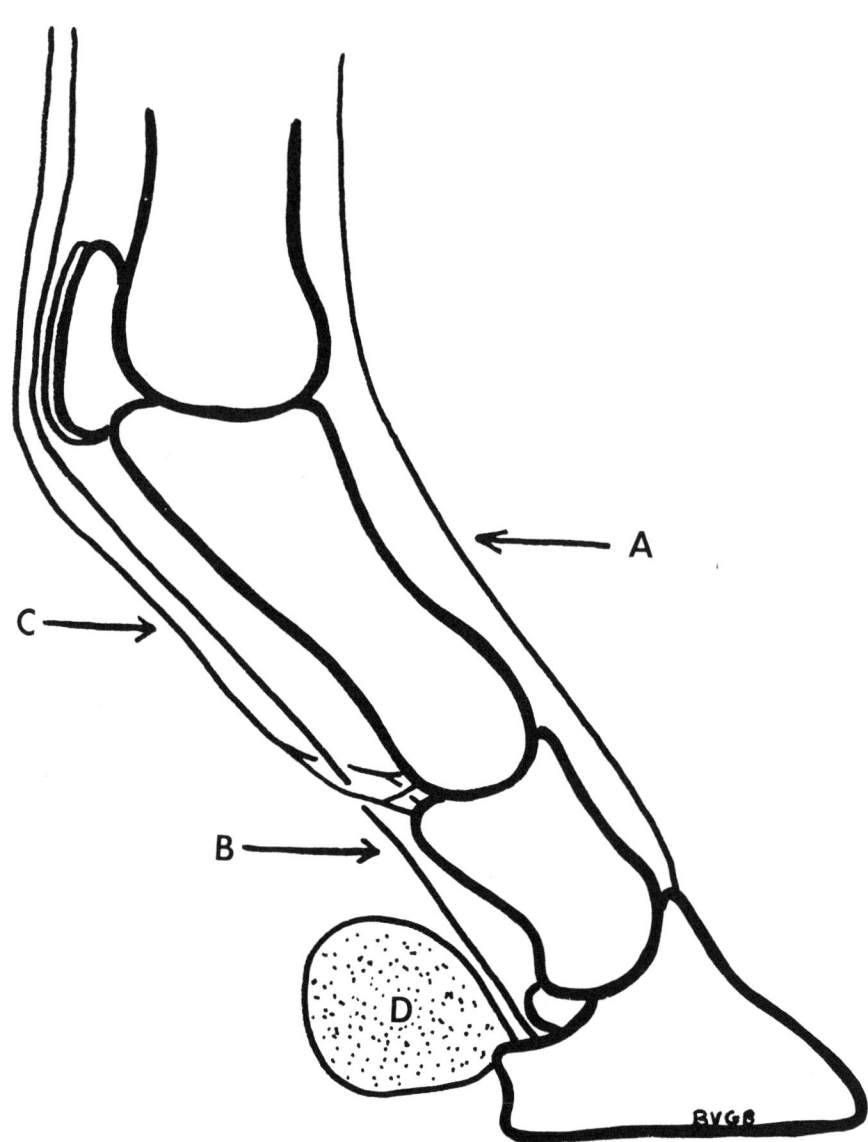

FIGURE 2. Distal Thoracic Limb: A–Common Digital Extensor Muscle Tendon; B–Deep Digital Flexor Muscle Tendon; C–Superficial Digital Flexor Muscle Tendon; D–Lateral Cartilage.

coffin joint which is "buried" underneath the hoof wall, (hence the name coffin). There is another small bone located at the back of the coffin joint called the *distal sesamoid* ("navicular") *bone*. The coffin bone is shaped roughly like the hoof and is involved in the condition called founder.

Three major muscle tendons attach to the bones of the inner foot and cause the foot to move, and all three of these muscles start in the region of the forearm. Along the front of the leg is a muscle called the *common digital extensor* which attaches to the front of the distal phalanx (coffin bone). When this muscle works it does several things, straightening up the knee and pulling each phalanx (the two pastern bones and the coffin bone) into a more forward position. In the horse this occurs just before the moving animal steps on his foot. The *deep digital flexor* sits close to bone along the back part of the leg, passing behind the navicular bone and attaching to the back of the coffin bone. When this muscle works the horse bends his knee and folds his foot up underneath himself as when first picking up his leg. A third muscle, the *superficial digital flexor* is located in the back of the leg just behind the deep digital flexor. This muscle attaches to both the long and short pastern bones and not the coffin bone, and must therefore split and pass around the deep digital flexor tendon. The superficial digital flexor muscle serves the same function as the deep digital flexor although it cannot help turn the coffin bone because it does not extend that far. These tendons play major roles in the conditions of contracted tendons, navicular disease, founder, and in deep cuts in the area. The *lateral cartilages* are pieces of cartilage (a sturdy structure not quite as hard as bone) which attach to the inside and outside of the coffin bone. These project up and back, looking somewhat like wings, to fill much of the side of the hoof, and they can actually be felt on a horse just above the side of the hoof wall toward the back. Sometimes these lateral cartilages partially change to bone, resulting in the condition known as sidebones.

The coffin bone is covered by a tissue called *periosteum*, ("around bone"). The periosteum contains numerous nerves and is very sensitive to pain.

Cover all of the above foot structures with skin (much as a mitten covers a hand), change it a little here and there, and the result is the hoof. At the top of the foot the skin gets thicker and looses its hair, a line called the *coronary band*. Below the coronary band is the *hoof wall*, again just a slightly changed type of skin. The hoof wall grows from the coronary band just as your fingernail grows from the base of

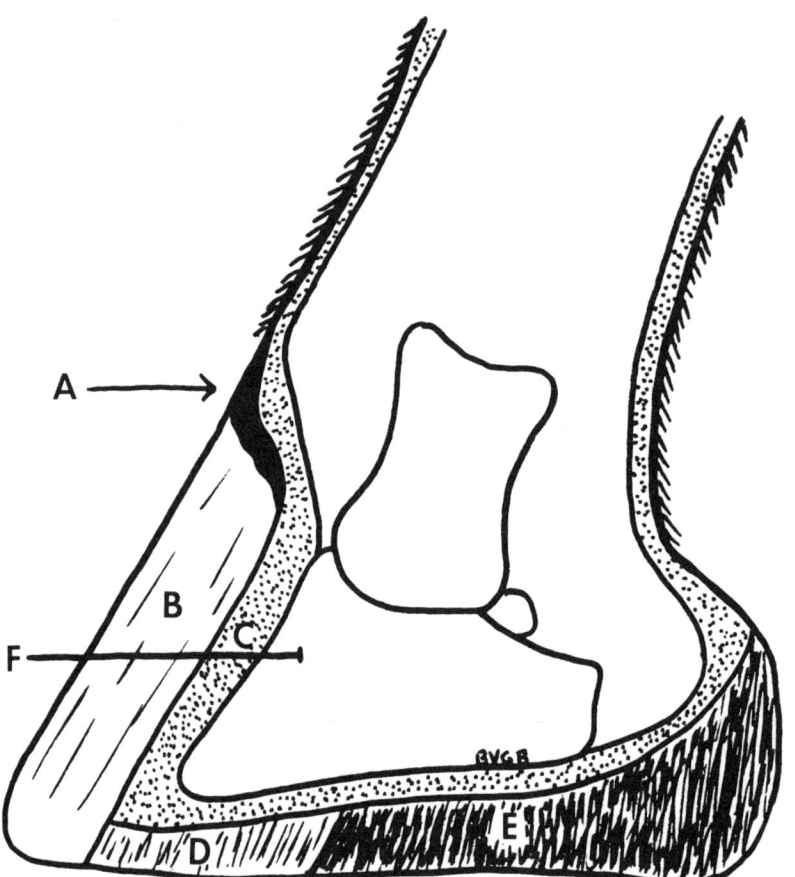

FIGURE 3. **The Hoof: A–Coronary Band; B–Hoof Wall; C–Periosteum; D–Sole; E–Frog; F–Incision Line for fig. 4.**

the nail. The inside of the hoof wall sits right next to the periosteum.

The "skin" which covers the bottom of the foot is also modified to help the horse. Part of it, the *sole*, is flat and hard. The *frog*, a "V"-shaped structure at the back, is softer and serves to cushion the inner structures when the horse is moving. (The horse walks like we do in that he lands on the heel first, then full foot, and pushes off with his toe.) The frog also attaches to a continuation of the periosteum.

The discussion thus far has dealt with the outer structures of the foot—the hoof wall, sole, and frog. The coverings of the inner structures that are held in place by attachment to the periosteum of the bone or its continuation. If the bottom half of the foot is cut off parallel to the ground we can obtain a closer look at how the hoof wall is held to the sensitive periosteum. The inside of the hoof wall was described by John Stump of Purdue University as being lined by major columns of projections pointing toward the coffin bone. From the coffin bone periosteum are similiar columns that fit snugly between the hoof wall columns, locking together. These major columns also have minor hoof wall columns projecting from them to give an even tighter fit. This fact becomes very important in the condition of founder.

We assume a foal is born with all the bones and muscles it will need as an adult, but we cannot assume that these structures will develop in a fashion to permit their most efficient use. That is what conformation is all about.

In discussing conformation several basic principles which hold true for both front and rear limbs should be considered. These will enable us to understand why certain conformations are more desirable than

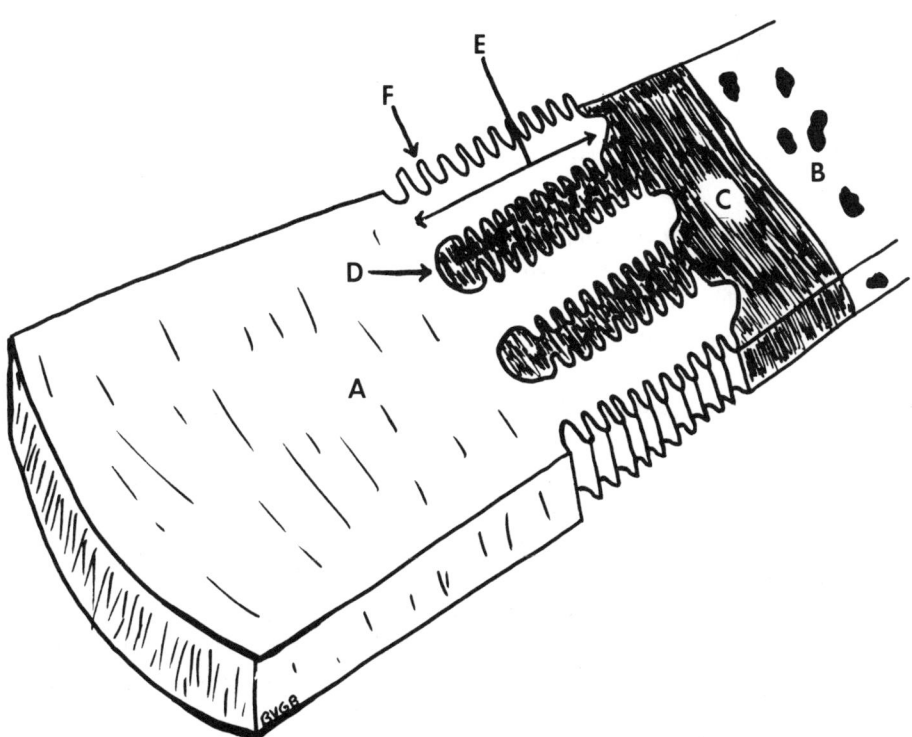

FIGURE 4. **Cross Section of the Hoof: A–Hoof Wall; B–Coffin Bone; C–Periosteum; D–Periosteal Column; E–Major Hoof Wall Column; F–Minor Hoof Wall Column.**

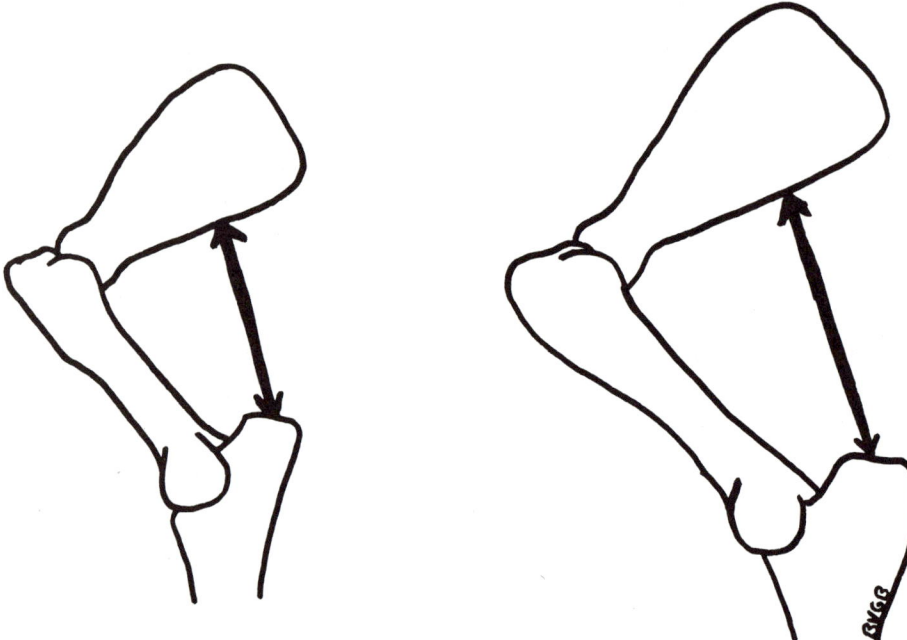

FIGURE 5. **Bone Length Affects Muscle Length.**

others. The number one principle is that while there is no such thing as an ideal conformation, there is one which is most efficient. The purpose for which the horse was intended will determine what is best. To put it another way, the conformation of the horse will determine its best use.

Bone size is proportional to muscle size. This statement becomes obvious when we consider that bone is living tissue which changes to match the demands of the body. A heavy muscle structure needs a heavy bone structure so that a sudden muscle contraction won't break the bone. A slender muscle certainly would not put as strong a demand on a bone, and thus the bone is finer. In addition, a long bone requires a long muscle to reach its entire length. Muscle strength is the result of muscle diameter. Are there many finely built draft horses? Similiarily, muscle action depends on muscle length. Five-gaited horses are not built like draft horses.

The power and shock absorption of a limb can be represented as the ratio between the fully extended length of the limb and its normal standing length. To illustrate this principle, stand with your knees stiff and jump as high as you can without bending them. Now bend your knees and try again. The first posture allowed the straightening of your leg only at the ankle, a situation similar to a horse with a straight shoulder or stifle. The second posture permitted a greater jump because there were bends to straighten at both the knee and ankle. Another contrast is to jump off a step first normally and then stiff-legged.

In discussing conformation of the forelimb each bone or region and respective "ideal" conformation for peak efficiency should be considered. The scapula has several functions including weight support, concussion absorption when moving, propulsion in turns, and maintenance of the center of gravity. The latter function helps prevent the horse from riding like a jack rabbit. A long scapula allows for a long muscle to the point of the elbow, and for better leverage by that muscle at the shoulder joint. In order to obtain this preferred length, the scapula must be at an angle of forty-five degrees to the ground, which is fairly easy to estimate by using the spine of the scapula as a landmark. To explain the stated forty-five degrees consider that a given horse has a definite size, thus limiting the verticle height of the

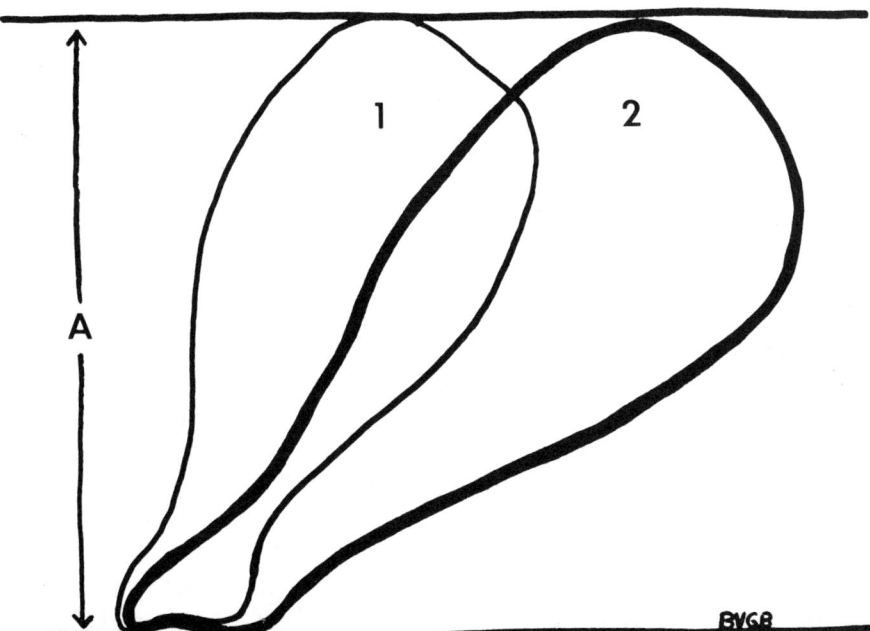

FIGURE 6. **Angulation of the Scapula.**

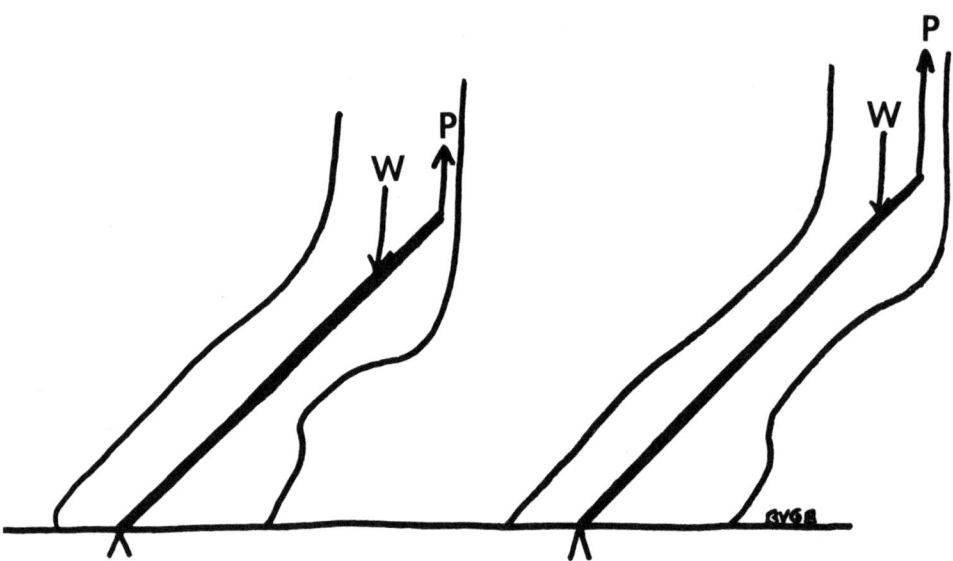

FIGURE 7. **The Foot as a Lever: P–Power of Muscle Tendons; W–Weight of the Body.**

scapula (seen as distance A, fig. 6). Scapula 1 is set a sixty degrees to the horizontal, and is noticeably shorter than scapula 2 at forty-five degrees. Angles much smaller than forty-five degrees cause the scapula to become so long as to result in disfiguration of the other limb bones.

The humerus should also have length to allow the muscles behind the shoulder joint and those which flex the elbow to have length. A ninety degrees angle between the scapula and the humerus allows for the greatest length to both bones without loss of muscle power.

Length in the radius and ulna is desirable for action of the knees and feet, as the muscles that work these areas begin here. Long cannon bones (metacarpals) will also help the length of the muscles going to the feet.

Much of the initial concussion of landing in a stride is absorbed in the area of the fetlock and below, and an intricate system of ligaments has been established to counteract this. During a race, the horse's fetlock often touches the ground when his foot first lands. Perfect alignment of the bones in this area occurs at the angle of forty-five degrees in the ideal horse. This permits greatest shock absorption with minimum wear and tear on ligaments and muscle tendons.

In the pastern area the ideal length of bone can vary. Long bones permit a longer stride and flexion of the area when the horse lands, for a smoother ride. But, it takes more effort on the part of the horse to work this type of foot. This build is ideal for racehorses. Compare the above to the foot of a horse that must work for long time periods. The extra energy required by the muscles to lift up the fetlock (the digital flexor muscles) would be too demanding, so shorter pastern bones would be more desirable. The accompanying illustration compares the two types of feet to levers. Note that the longer pastern (lever) would take more power *(P)* to lift the same body weight *(W)*.

In motion, as the front limb lands the leg muscles are responsible for moving the body forward, not for moving the limb back. Good conformation allows the horse to do this without putting unnecessary stress and strain on bones, muscles, tendons, and ligaments. It permits the most efficient use of body parts, which means muscles use less energy to do the job, which means it takes less oats to provide this energy, which means a money savings to you (not to mention less manure to shovel). Smoothness of motion is comparable to the follow-through of a ball player and permits less energy waste. The choppiness of the "pony trot" is not only hard to ride, it is also inefficient.

The front of the horse has two factors affecting shock absorption. These forelimbs are attached to the bones of the body only by muscle, not by bone. These muscles can then absorb some of the shock of movement, instead of sending it on to the bones of the body. The amount of angle at the shoulder, elbow, and fetlock joints aids in shock absorption, as well as in power output. Remember the difference between jumping off a step with stiff knees and with knees bent.

Looking at a well made horse from the front, the scapula should join the humerus at a slight angle, and a line drawn from the shoulder, through the elbow, knee, fetlock, and foot should be straight. This indicates that the joints can move straight forward and back and that no stress is placed on the ligaments. Horses that toe-out put added stress on the inside of all the involved joints, and if worked too hard could become lame. The outer structures are stressed if the animal toes-in.

Occasionally the scapulas (shoulder blades) are positioned too far forward on the chest, which is narrower in the front than it is along the sides. As the limb moves straight forward and back, the scapula must be far enough out along the chest so that the elbows don't hit the ribs. If the scapula is too far forward, the animal must compensate by turning the elbows away from the body ("out at the elbows"), putting

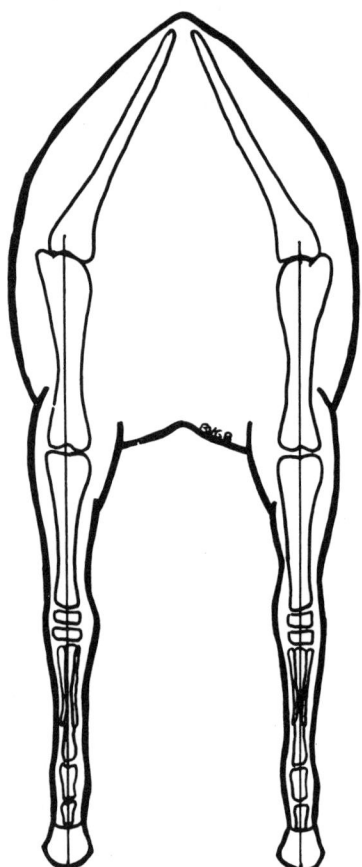

FIGURE 8. **Front View of the Thoracic Limbs.**

excessive strain on the inside of that joint. Some of these horses will also walk with their toes pointed in. A second complication of the poorly positioned scapula is very apparent when the horse moves. Watching the animal from the front, we see the left foot land toward the right of the center line of travel and the right foot land to the left, sort of like the horse in the movie "Cat Ballou" that couldn't walk a straight line. As shown, A is normal with each limb traveling almost straight forward, while the body of B must weave from side to side to travel straight forward. Imagine the positions of the elbows and feet of horse B. This is obviously not an efficient way to travel, and results in extra strain to the ligaments on the outside of the limb.

Variations from normal conformation, injuries, and internal prob-

Equine Shock Absorbers · 27

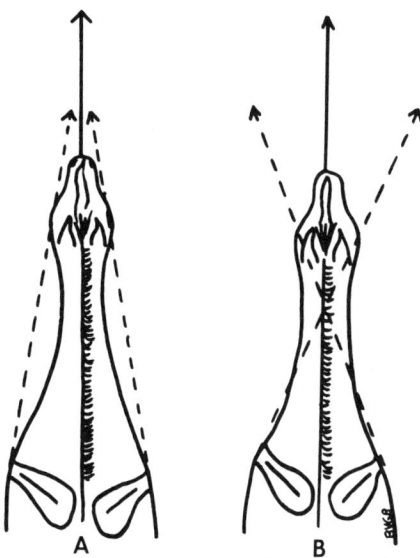

FIGURE 9. **Top View of a Horse:**
⟶ –Direction of Travel
- ⟶ –Direction of Limb Motion

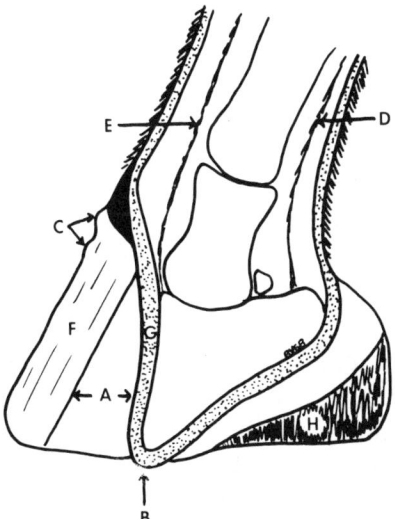

FIGURE 10. **Foot with Laminitis:** A–Separation of Hoof Wall and Periosteum; B–Protrusion of Coffin Bone and Periosteum through the Sole; C–Abnormal New Hoof Growth; D–Deep Digital Flexor Muscle Tendon; E–Common Digital Extensor Muscle Tendon; F–Hoof Wall; G–Periosteum; H–Frog.

lems can result in any of a number of pathologic conditions in the forelimb. Two of these deserve special mention because of their frequency and severity in the horse.

Laminitis literally means "inflammation of the lamina of the hoof," the lamina being the major and minor columns described previously under the anatomy of the foot. The horse has 600 major columns and about 100,000 minor columns holding the hoof wall to the periosteum. In laminitis, there is a separation of the columns of the hoof wall from the columns of the periosteum. The deep digital flexor muscle, attached to the back of the coffin bone, is stronger than the common digital extensor muscle in front, causing the back of the coffin bone to rotate up and the toe of the coffin bone down. The coffin bone is then no longer parallel to the hoof wall. The resulting pressure of the bone on the sole can cause the toe to push the sole down or to push a hole through the sole. Additionally, the blood supply to the growth area of the hoof wall (just inside the coronary band) is disturbed, and results in either an abnormal new hoof wall including circular rings, or in the actual loss of the hoof wall.

There are several situations that can result in laminitis, some more common than others. Overeating disease was one of the first names applied to this condition and it remains a primary cause. Horses that have access to large quantities of grain, whether as a daily ration or as an unplanned trip into the feed room, will find themselves in trouble. One of the substances that grain digests into is a *toxin* ("poison") that in enough quantity will produce laminitis.

Water founder is a second form of laminitis. Overheated horses that drink large amounts of cold water often develop the problem.

Horses will road founder from the concussion or beating of the feet on hard surfaces, especially for long periods of time or at a fast speed. This type of laminitis is usually seen in unconditioned horses and in ones with thin walls and soles.

Good green clover and alfalfa pastures can cause problems. For some reason overweight horses, especially ones with fat cresty necks, are more apt to grass founder than others, thus explaining the higher incidence of it seen in Shetland and Welsh ponies. This condition is occasionally seen during the winter in horses fed alfalfa or clover hay.

Mares that have foaled or aborted a foal may develop postparturient laminitis, a very serious form. Usually this type of founder is due to the mare retaining a portion of the fetal membranes and/or developing a uterine infection. Some mares refounder after each foal is born or when carrying a foal, while other old foundered mares actually show a definite improvement while pregnant.

Other causes of laminitis are as numerous as the words in this book, but include an abnormal reaction to a drug or to generalized infections. One cause of laminitis should be stressed: ANY TIME A HORSE RUNS A HIGH FEVER, LAMINITIS CAN RESULT. Be sure to get help immediately!

What signs are shown by foundered horses? Usually the front feet are affected, although occasionally all four are involved. The standing position changes drastically because weight is shifted to the nonpainful hind legs, which are tucked forward under the body. The front legs carry as little weight as possible and are positioned further forward than normal. The horse is in pain and is very reluctant to move. It is often possible to feel increased warmth in the region of the foot.

The best first aid for suspected founder is an *immediate* call to your veterinarian, in addition to stopping the cause (get the horse out of the oats, away from the fresh grass), standing the horse in cold water or mud, or applying ice packs on the feet until professional help arrives.

The outlook is not too good for the foundered horse. Remember that as many as 60 million major and minor columns have pulled loose from each other. What are the odds that all of these can return back into normal position? Less severely foundered animals can return to near normal and with careful diet, hoof care, and special shoeing can be useful. Caution must be used because these horses seem to founder easily a second time. Most severe cases have little hope. Many veterinary researchers are studying laminitis and some of their findings look promising, but none have yet proven to be consistently effective. The best treatment for founder is still the prevention of it.

Navicular disease is another of the uncurable lamenesses. Unfortunately, while the pathology of the foot is well known the cause of the pathology is still speculation.

The navicular (distal sesamoid) bone is a small structure located at the back of the coffin joint with the tendon of the deep digital flexor muscle running behind it. The function of this small bone is to protect the tendon as it crosses the coffin joint by giving it a smooth surface to slide across.

Concussion is described as the most probable cause of navicular disease. The front legs are used by the horse for landing, the push of the stride coming from the hind legs. Horses that perform strenuously, in racing, jumping, cutting, and barrel racing, are affected more by this condition, with performance on rough or hard surfaces greatly increasing concussion. (Try jumping up and down fifty times on a sidewalk and fifty times on a lawn.) Upright conformation (straight pasterns) puts more abnormal stress on this small bone, as does the trimming of a horse with upright pasterns by taking off too much in the heels.

A horse with navicular disease is usually slightly lame on a front foot but gets better when rested. If worked hard he is very lame the next day. This may go on for several months until the animal is almost constantly lame. Other things can cause the lameness described and a positive diagnosis may be difficult, requiring radiographs (X-rays) and anesthesia of the nerves to the foot.

For any of several reasons there is excess wear and concussion on the navicular bone, which causes the side next to the deep digital flexor tendon to become rough. This rough surface tears at the flexor tendon as it slides across the bone, causing pain. Ligaments holding the navicular bone in place also receive rough use, and these become painful when moved by other bones. Although the horse shows lameness in one front foot, both feet are affected because both have the same conformation and take the same beating.

There is NO cure for navicular disease. In some horses the pain from the condition can be stopped by cutting the nerves that go to the bone, but these nerves also go to the horse's heels. Thus injury, such as a nail into the heel, would go unnoticed unless the animal was watched carefully. The horse could not feel the back of its foot when it stepped down and thus would be unsafe for riding, especially on uneven ground. Other problems can occur from cutting the nerves to the foot, and hopefully your veterinarian will never have to explain them to you.

Butazolidin is the drug most frequently given to lame horses to mask the pain of lameness. I can appreciate that a lame horse at a show is a "minor emergency" to those who want to show it, but I think we should take a closer look at this drug.

Butazolidin is a pain killer, many times more powerful than asprin. In fact, it is so powerful that some horses with broken legs don't even notice the pain they are in! Can you imagine what would happen to a horse with a broken leg if it was given "Bute" to hide the lameness so it could "go in one more pleasure class," or "run the barrels today because the owners have driven so far to come to the show," or "run in this race because I just know he can win"? You wouldn't believe the excuses some people come up with! Several years ago a man came up to me on the sly at one of the state fairs, asking if I had any "Bute." When asked why he wanted it, he took me to his stall and showed me his top halter stallion. The horse would not put any weight on its left hind leg. He said the horse was in a trailer accident on the way to the fair and had hurt its leg. It was obvious to any observer that the stifle was severely bruised. He wanted some Butazolidin so the horse could show in halter that afternoon. I said I did have some and that I would be glad to give the horse some *AFTER* I sent the veterinarian's release for that horse to the horse show office. The owner didn't like that idea at all and went off to find another source of the drug. A horse in the condition of this stallion could easily have broken off a piece of bone near that stifle or torn several ligaments or muscles. Pain is nature's way of protecting that leg. I would never ask a family member to perform with a condition like that and I certainly wouldn't ask it of my animals either.

Butazolidin does have a place in helping lame horses, but decisions for its use should be made by a veterinarian. Only in cases where the animal will not be hurt by its use is there justification for giving it, and then only when the animal's handler is the type of person who will follow directions! If the veterinarian says the horse can safely be used for pleasure, the handler should not also then put it in reining and barrels. Rules of the association that govern the show or race will often determine if the drug can be used, and that decision must be abided by. It was established for the good of the animal not for the benefit of some point-hungry or purse-happy horse owner or trainer. When used properly, Butazolidin is a valuable tool to have. When used improperly, it is dangerous at best.

2
"P" Is for Push and Pelvic Limb (The Pelvic Limb)

In a discussion of the ability of a horse to travel properly it is essential to also understand the basic anatomy of the pelvic (hind) limb.

Bone structure starts with the pelvis, which is actually a junction of six bones, three per side. The *ilium* is the most forward of these and is seen externally at the area we call the *tuber coxae* ("point of the hip"). Attached to this are most of the *gluteal muscles*. These give the rounded appearance to the hip and are important in rearing and in giving the powerful push during motion, especially in the gallop or in the jump. The *ischium* is the farthest-back bone of the three, seen as the *ischiatic tuberosity* ("point of the croup"), and used as a guide when talking about the length of the hip (distance from the point of the hip to the point of the croup). It is to the ischium that the powerful muscles at the back of the limb attach, the ones we look at to determine the width of the stifle and the amount of inner muscling hidden by the tail. The third bone, the *pubis*, forms the front edge of the bottom of the pelvis to which the abdominal muscles attach. In addition to the prominences mentioned, there are two holes in the pelvis called the *obturator foramen*. Through these pass nerves going to the muscles on the inside of the leg to prevent the horse from doing a sideward split. Pressure on one of these nerves (as during foaling) can cause a paralysis of these muscles, hopefully only temporary. These inner muscles belong to the adductor group which attach at the area where

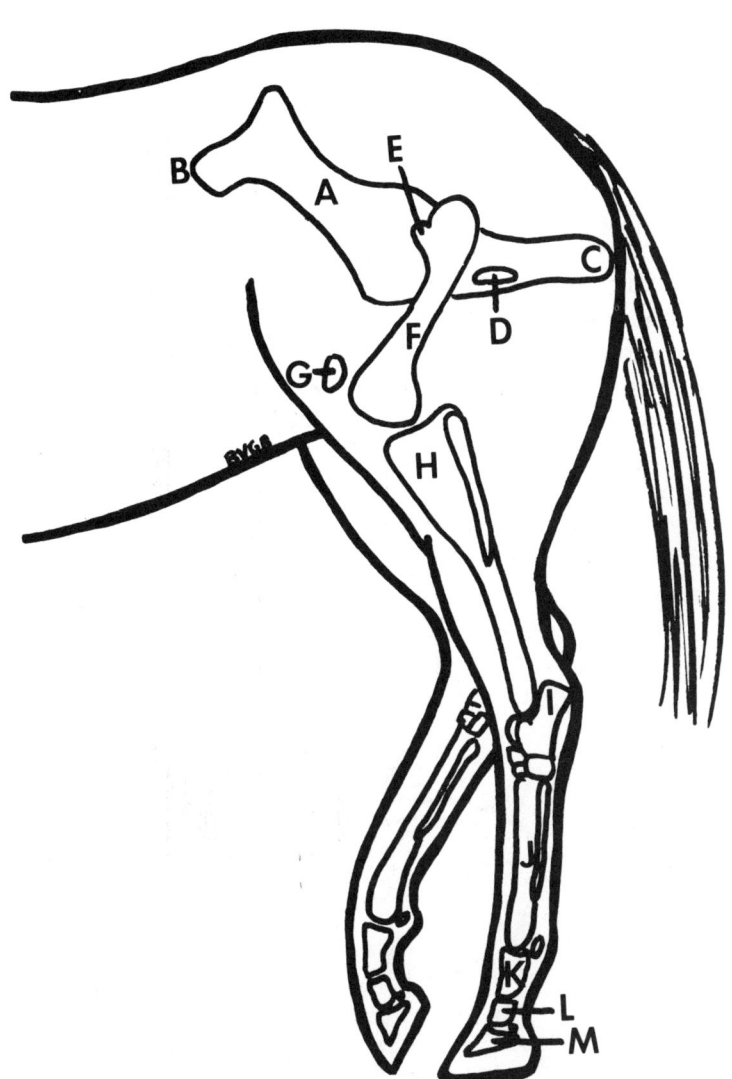

FIGURE 11. **Bones of the Pelvic Limb:** A–Ilium; B–Tuber Coxae; C–Ischiatic Tuberosity; D–Obturator Foramen; E–Hip Joint; F–Femur; G–Patella; H–Tibia; I–Point of the Hock; J–Metatarsal Bone; K–Proximal Phalanx; L–Middle Phalanx; M–Distal Phalanx.

34 • Your Horse's Health

the right and left halves of the pelvis join. The region where the three bones on each side come together is demarcated by a crater-looking structure called the *acetabulum*. It is this cup shape that forms the socket of the hip joint.

The other half of the hip joint is formed by the head of the *femur* ("thigh bone"), which is rounded much like a ball. The *hip joint* of the horse is basically a ball-and-socket joint with the rounded head of the femur fitting into the cup-shaped acetabulum of the pelvis. In man, upright posture and the angle at which the femur meets the pelvis allow the body weight to help hold the two bones together. In the horse the two bones meet at nearly a right angle, so body weight doesn't help the equine. Nature has provided two strong ligaments to overcome this disadvantage, as is seen in an exaggerated form in figure 13–B.

In front of the femur is a group of large muscles that straighten the *stifle joint* by attaching first to the *patella* ("kneecap"), and then to the front edge of the *tibia*, the main bone just below the stifle. The horse is the only animal which can sleep standing up. In order for this to occur several ligaments, tendons, and other unique structures must be

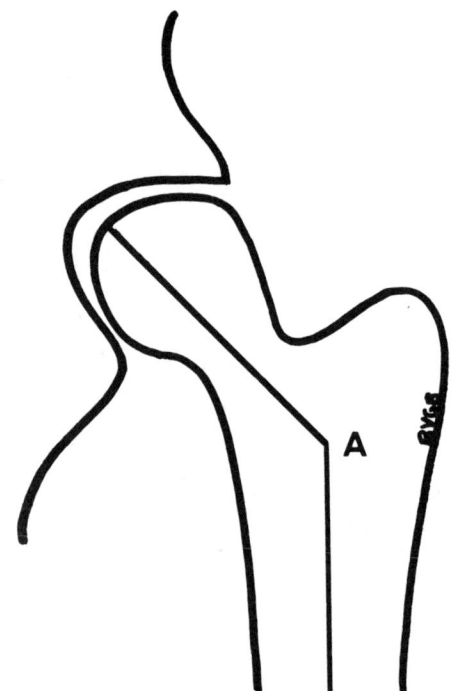

FIGURE 12. **Human Hip Joint: A–Angle of the Hip.**

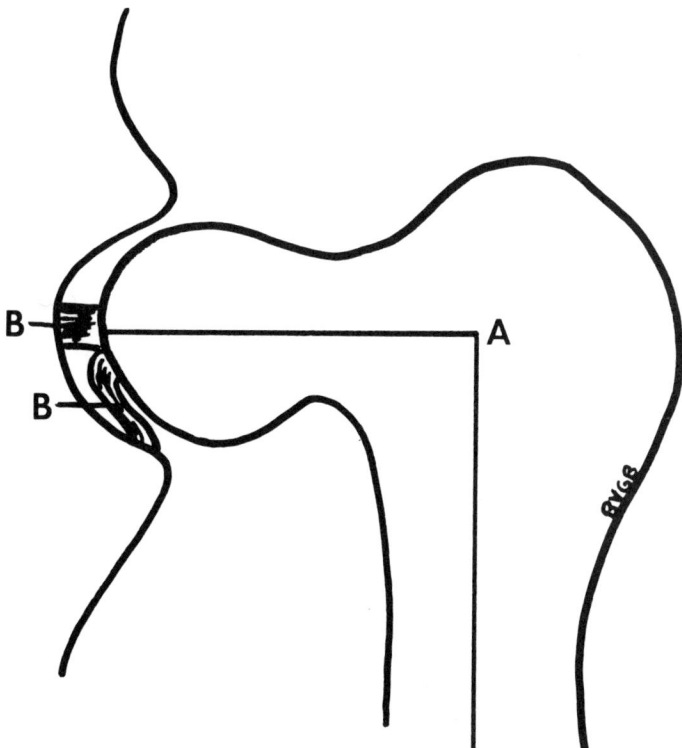

FIGURE 13. **Horse Hip Joint: A–Angle of the Hip; B–Ligaments of the Hip.**

present so that when the muscles go to sleep the horse won't fall down. As part of this arrangement, the stifle, can be voluntarily locked into a position for rest and then voluntarily unlocked for movement.

On the front of the femur at the bottom end is the groove in which the patella ("kneecap") slices. The inside edge of this groove forms a large ridge in the horse. A good-sized muscle attaches at the top of the patella, and three ligaments attach the bottom of the patella to the tibia. This muscle normally pulls the patella up and down in the groove. When the horse locks the stifle this muscle works harder to pull the patella higher and then a muscle on the inside of the leg pulls the patella toward the inside of the leg, over the top of the large ridge. When both muscles relax the patella remains hooked on top of the ridge and the stifle is "fixed." When the horse no longer wants to rest he uses the large muscle to pull the patella up, and another muscle on the outside of the leg pulls the patella back into normal alignment with the groove. These muscles now relax.

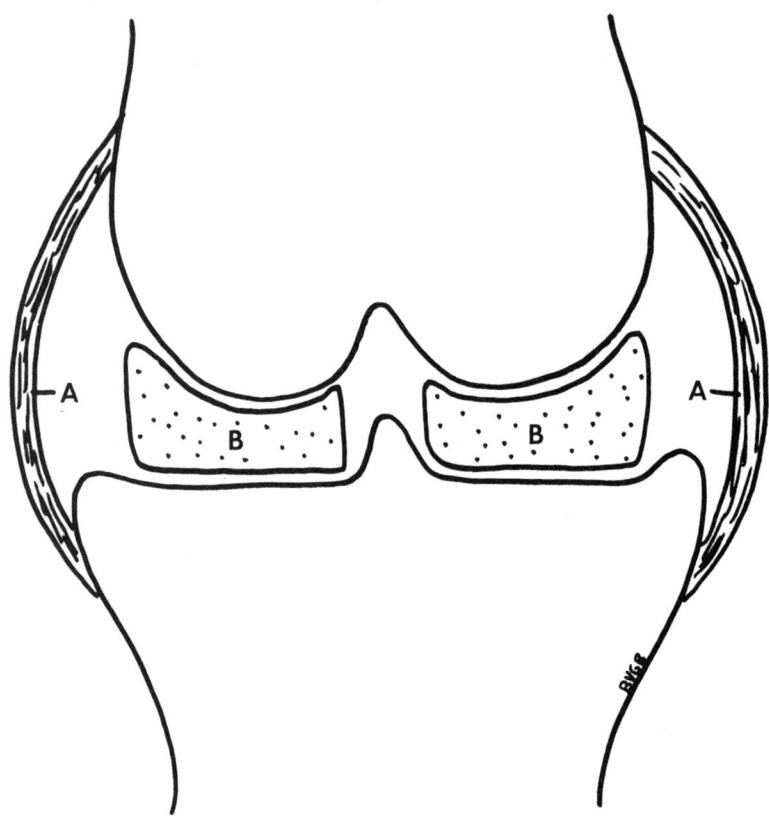

FIGURE 14. **Stifle Joint, Front View: A–Collateral Ligaments; B–Menisci.**

The tibia and a small bone, the *fibula*, are located in the true leg, crus, or gaskin region. All the muscles which work the lower limb start at the top of this region. The *gastrocnemius muscle* (which represents our "calf" muscle) is the largest of this group and attaches on the *point of the hock*.

The *tarsal* ("hock") *joint*, which corresponds to the human ankle, usually has six small bones. One of these, the *calcanean* or fibular *tarsal bone*, sticks out behind to form the point of the hock.

Below the hock the three *metatarsal bones* form the cannon bone and the two smaller splint bones. In front of two *sesamoid bones* at the fetlock, the metatarsals meet the *proximal phalanx* ("long pastern"), which in turn meets the *middle phalanx* ("short pastern") at the pastern joint. Just below the top of the hoof is the *coffin joint*, where the *distal phalanx* ("coffin bone") joins the rest of the limb.

The stifle is a real mechanical marvel and deserves a special description. Two structures, specifically designed to stabilize the joint, are called *collateral ligaments*. These attach to the outside of the joint, one per side, to prevent the tibia from moving to the right or left of the femur above it. In the space between the two bones nature has placed two wedges of cartilage, the *menisci*. The bottom of the femur is rounded, while the top of the tibia is flat. Consider a well-aired tire on a road, in which there is minimal contact between the tire and the ground—one-point contact. This is painful if it is bone to bone. A flat tire has a lot of surface contact with the road, and therefore spreads the weight above over a much larger surface. In the body, the menisci are rounded on top and flat on the bottom to spread the weight

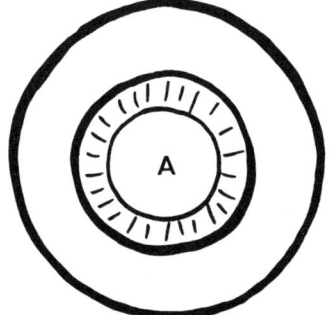 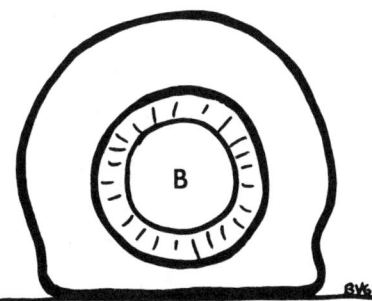

FIGURE 15. **Types of Surface Contact: A–Inflated Tire; B–Flat Tire.**

evenly on the top of the tibia, as does the flat tire. Two other ligaments are associated with the stifle, and their actions are best described from a side view. One *cruciate ligament* prevents the tibia from moving forward to the femur, while the second prevents the tibia from moving too far behind the femur.

The function of the hind limb differs from that of the front because it serves as a power generator, not as a primary shock absorber. This very important function also requires correct conformation, and all the basic principles described for the thoracic limb also hold true here.

The primary consideration for shock absorption was that maximum angulation at the joints be present. This is the same type of angulation which permits maximum power. Consider again standing flat footed and jumping off a step or ledge without bending your knees compared to jumping with knees bent.

From a side view the pelvis can be set in any of several positions depending on the purpose of the animal. The most efficient pelvic slope

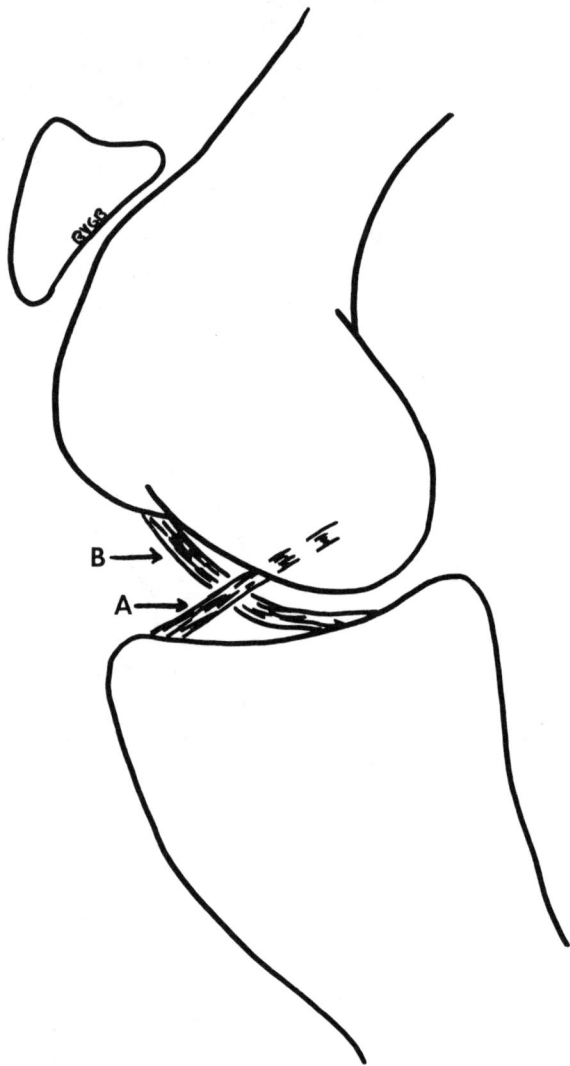

FIGURE 16. **Stifle Joint, Side View: A–Cranial Cruciate Ligament; B–Caudal Cruciate Ligament.**

is a thirty degree angle from the horizon. The pelvic part of the hip joint, the acetabulum, limits how far back the limb can go because of its cup shape. At thirty degrees the horse has a large angle for pushing off but yet maintains the ability to work with his feet under him. If the slope is greater than thirty degrees, we see a steep external slope to the rump. A horse with this type of conformation works with his feet under him and often is a heavier-muscled individual. Limits to the backward phase of the stride caused by the position of the acetabulum prevent normal amount of length to the stride in the steep rumped individual. Extreme examples of this type include the cutting horse and the draft horse. In the individual with a flat croup, the pelvis is less than thirty degrees, resulting in abilities opposite to those just described. The flat croup, so desirable in the Arabian and Saddlebred, allows the horse to have maximum length to the stride but tends to minimize the maneuverability afforded when the legs are underneath. Training and other conformation factors can influence either of these natural tendencies.

The "ideal" position for the femur is forty-five degrees from the horizontal, or vertical. Maximum muscle length provides maximum length for contraction, is more efficient, and therefore is more desirable. A forty-five degree position for the femur gives length to the powerful muscles which attach at the back edge of the pelvis and run to near the stifle joint. These are important in the push of the stride, so length is very desirable.

Maximum angulation, without overdoing to the point where advantages are lost, is achieved when the tibia meets the femur at an angle of ninety degrees. As a result, the tibia can have maximum length for its allowable space. Muscles which run the length of the tibia work the stifle, hock, and feet, and because these are such important joints for power, it is essential to have the long muscles here. As the stifle joint gets straighter in conformation, the muscles in the region get shorter, and in straight-legged individuals these muscles are therefore less effective. This conformation is a very real trend in many American Quarter Horses today.

If long bones are bred for, without angulation, the natural tendency would be for the horses to become taller. Since this is not always what happens, something else must be taking place. As certain major bones increase in length, like the femur and tibia, others, like the cannon, shorten. Balance must be maintained.

The angle at the fetlock is slightly straighter than the similiar angle

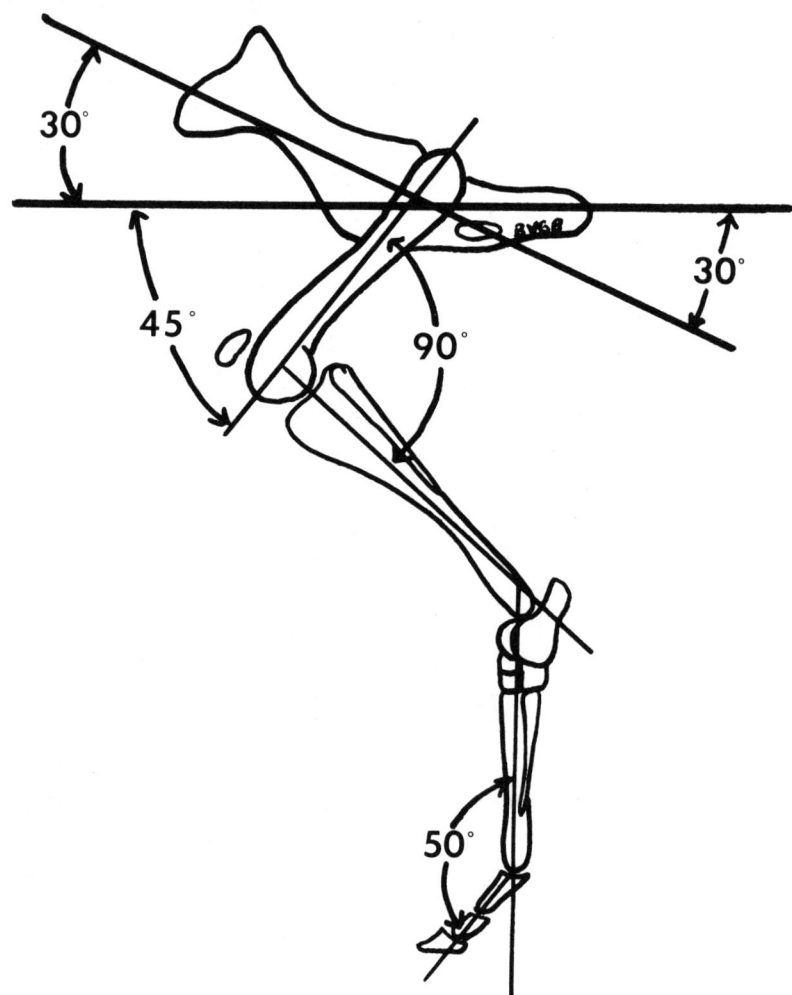

FIGURE 17. **Angulation of the Pelvic Limb.**

on the front limb. The fifty degree "ideal" angle permits less for shock absorption but may be more advantageous in propulsion.

A *"locked" stifle* is the most common problem in the rear limb of the horse, and it is one definitely related to conformation. From the side view, a horse with little angulation looks "postlegged" or "straight legged". These are the individuals which tend to have stifle problems. A "stifled" horse has a patella that is in the locked position at times other than when the horse is resting. If the stifle is straight, with not enough angulation, the patella is carried too high because the muscle pulling it up is shortened. (Measure the distance from the top front of the thigh of your leg to just below the kneecap when your knee is straight. The distance, which represents muscle length, is longer with a bent knee. Since ligaments can't shorten, the muscle does.) If the patella rides too high it will more easily slip over the ridge and can "lock" while the animal is trying to walk.

Another situation which occurs in a straight-stifled horse is one where the horse is in training and is worked fairly hard. He is allowed to rest at night and the next morning can't bend one or both hind limbs. In this horse everything is normal during the work and rest. When he tries to unlock the patella the muscle that pulls it up is so tired, and perhaps stiff, from the exercise that it can't get enough strength to pull the kneecap up.

Problems with the stifles are very real, and so are problems involving the hock joint.

Three types of conditions involving the hock are termed spavins, but only two of these are severe. It is important to know the difference. *Blood spavin* is not a true pathologic condition. A large vein, the *medial saphenous*, courses up the inside of the horse's leg. Many people never notice this vein until the animal is lame and figure that because they hadn't noticed it before, it must now be causing the lameness. This large vessel is normal.

Bog spavin is a distention of the hock joint by a large amount of fluid, similar to what happens with a severely sprained ankle. Although nutritional deficiencies can result in bog spavin, the usual cause is a combination of poor conformation and hard use. A horse with straight hocks takes a lot of pounding on joint surfaces because the leg lacks the angles necessary for proper shock absorption. Add to that the stress placed on the joint by fast stops and turns asked of many horses. The resulting damage to the delicate membrane which encloses the joint, the *joint capsule,* causes it to produce an increased amount of synovial, or joint fluid. This results in the swellings seen on the inside front of

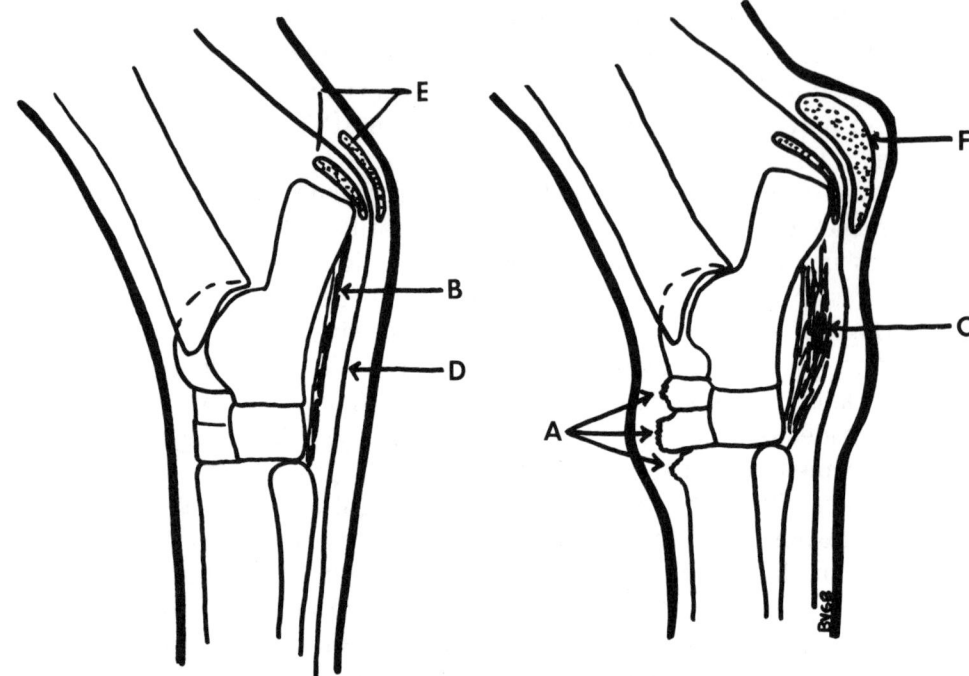

FIGURE 18. **Normal and Abnormal Hocks: A–Bone Spavin; B–Plantar Ligament; C–Curb; D–Superficial Digital Flexor Muscle Tendon; E–Bursas of the Superficial Digital Flexor Muscle Tendon; F–Capped Hock.**

the hock and to either side of the back of the hock, below the point.

Bone spavin is the second severe form of spavin, with conformation again playing a major role in the development of this condition. Sickle-hock and cow-hock conformations predispose horses to bone spavin. These individuals also tend to have thin hocks. Stress, such as quick stops, and dietary deficiencies may also cause the development of this condition. The bones of the tarsus ("hock") are arranged in two irregular rows. In bone spavin, new excess bone grows on the inside front of the bones of the middle row of tarsal bones, the bottom row of tarsal bones, and/or the top of the cannon bone. As this bone grows it interferes with normal motion of the middle and bottom joints of the hock. This interference causes pain and lameness. With rest and time both joints may actually grow shut, becoming nonfunctional.

Curb is another condition affecting structures of the hock region. From the point of the hock to the top of the cannon bone a ligament, the *plantar ligament*, functions to help stabilize the back of the hock.

A swelling and thickening of this ligament produces a bump on the back side of the joint. Kicking trailer doors or stall walls and extreme action at this joint can cause the condition, especially in animals with sickle hocks or cow hocks.

Capped hock is a swelling at the point of the hock which is usually the result of the animal kicking out and hurting this structure. The tendon of a muscle crosses right over the point of the hock. To protect this tendon the horse has developed two *bursas* in the area. These structures, which are similar to small water-filled balloons, cushion the tendon from the bone and from external damage. Injuries to the point of the hock may result in a swelling of one or both bursas, creating the condition of capped hock.

Problems of the pelvic limb are very real for the horse. Proper conformation will eliminate most of them, another reason that the importance of conformation cannot be overemphasized.

3
A Column of Support (The Vertebral Column)

A feature of vital importance is the structure which holds the front and back halves of the body together—the *vertebral column*. The importance of this structure is much more significant, however, because it offers support and protection.

Disregarding the bones in the tail, the horse has thirty-six bones in the vertebral column, named for their location. The *cervical*, or neck area of any mammal contains seven vertebrae. This holds true whether the horse has a long thin neck or a short thick one, or whether the mammal is a giraffe or a human. The bone which is located next to the skull, the *atlas*, is shaped somewhat like a butterfly. As viewed by the rider, it helps form the shape of the neck just behind the ears.

The *axis*, or second cervical vertebrae, has a tall upper projection which serves as an important anchor for several ligaments and muscles. The remainder of the cervical bones are shaped in a "typical" pattern and include *spinous* and *transverse processes* and a *vertebral foramen*, through which the spinal cord runs.

There are eighteen *thoracic vertebrae* in the region of the chest, the largest number of any domestic animal. Associated with each of these bones is a pair of *ribs*, and thus the long athletic chest of the horse. Compared to the "typical" vertebra, a thoracic vertebra has a tall spinous process. Another difference is that the transverse processes are greatly reduced in size because the ribs serve the same function.

A Column of Support • 45

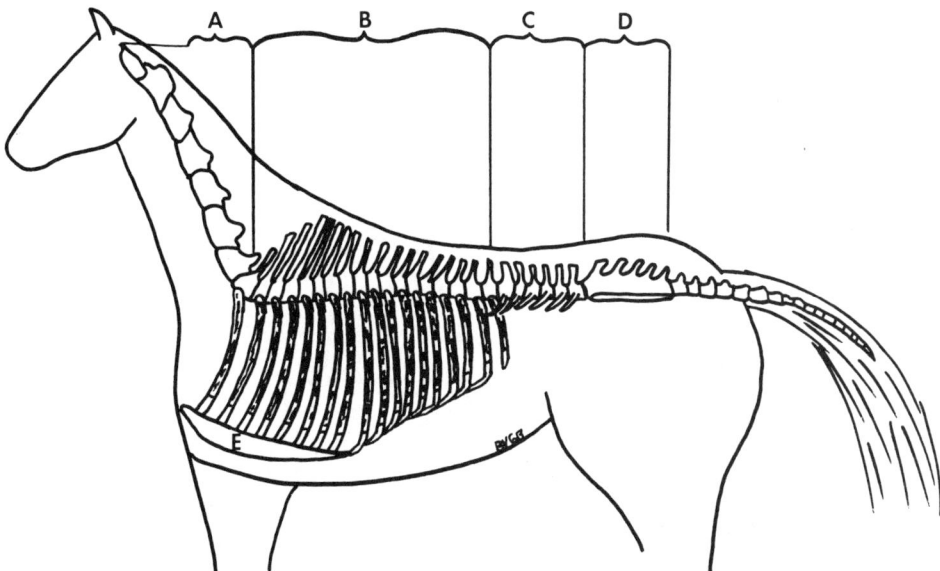

FIGURE 19. **Vertebral Column: A–Cervical Vertebrae; B–Thoracic Vertebrae; C–Lumbar Vertebrae; D–Sacral Vertebrae.**

Behind the thorax there are six *lumbar vertebrae* in the loin region. Each has exaggerated transverse processes which, with their associated muscle, give the needed width to the back while protecting vital abdominal structures. It is commonly said that the Arabian horse has one less lumbar vertebra and this accounts for its shorter back and tail set. According to the Arabian breed association, this is incorrect. There are six vertebrae, but each may be somewhat smaller than usual.

Between the two halves of the pelvis is the *sacrum*, a single bone formed by the fusion of five sacral vertebrae. The transverse processes are exaggerated to join to portions of the pelvis, forming the *sacroiliac joints*.

The vertebral column provides bony protection for the spinal cord throughout its length, helping to prevent bruising to the structure. In addition to support for the spinal cord, the column also offers support for the limbs and structures of the thorax and abdomen.

Ribs surround the vital structures of the chest cavity, supporting their position and protecting their function. Opposite the vertebral column, the *sternum* attaches to cartilages from the ribs to complete the rigid covering. Moving back along the chest, it can be observed

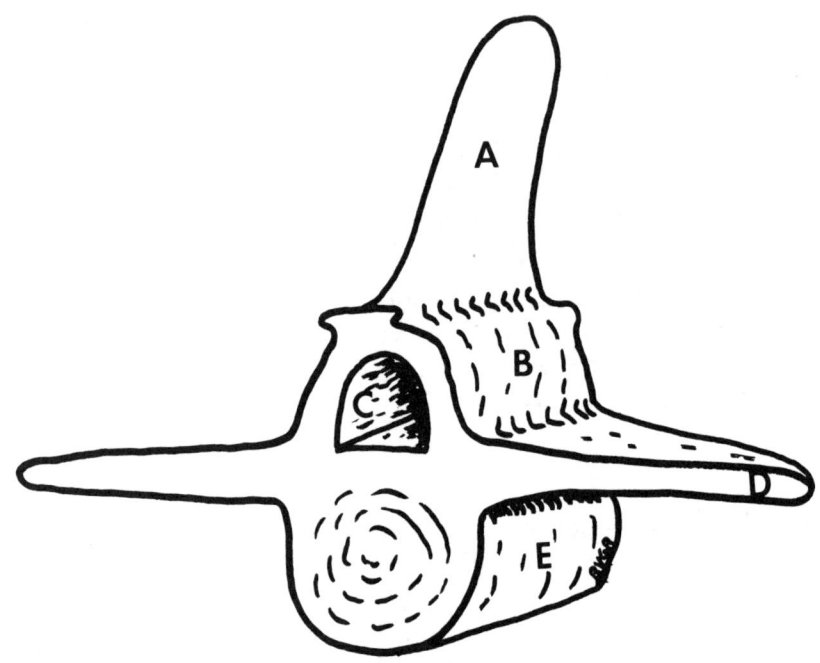

FIGURE 20. A "Typical" Vertebra: A–Spinous Process; B–Arch; C–Vertebral Foramen; D–Transverse Process; E–Body.

that each rib is slightly shorter than the one ahead of it. This helps create the appearance of the "athletic waist" described in horses.

4
The Anatomy of a Sigh (The Respiratory System)

The act of breathing is a marvelous feat accomplished by coordination of several muscles, nerves, blood vessels, and specific respiratory structures. One of the most obvious of these structures is the nose. All natural breathing in the horse must occur through the *nose*, a characteristic not true of other domestic animals. Odors are sensed at the back of the nose, near the level of the eye, and decisions are made whether the food smells acceptable or whether it has been contaminated by worming medicine. Most air passes the nasal area quickly, passing over the soft palate and the *epiglottis*, a piece of cartilage guarding the opening to the *trachea* ("windpipe"). Immediately behind the epiglottis is a specialized area of the trachea, the *larynx*, which consists of several pieces of cartilage. In humans the larynx forms an enlargement called the Adam's apple, or voice box. It also is the location of the *vocal folds* or cords which are responsible for sound in animals. On either side of the larynx a fold of tissue connects from the side to the bottom of the larynx, forming a "V". Muscles control the tightness of these vocal folds, and air movements cause them to vibrate. The result is voice of different pitches. Occasionally something happens to damage the nerve which supplies the muscles working one of the two vocal folds, resulting in a laxness to it. Air moving across the membrane causes it to move excessively, a condition called roaring.

As the trachea, a tube of many connected "C"-shaped cartilages, enters the thorax, it reaches a position above the heart and divides into two. The left *primary bronchus* goes into the left lung and the right goes to the two major portions of the right lung. The left lung of the horse has no lobes, unlike that of other animals, being one solid piece of tissue. The right lung only has one extra lobe, which fills the space behind the heart, in contrast to the four lobes seen in other animals. This accessory lobe, and the fact that the heart is located mainly on the left side, accounts for the fact that the right lung is larger than the left.

The lung tissue is filled with successively smaller channels which carry air to the final microscopic area, the *alveolus*. Within the millions of these little areas bordered by small branches of blood vessels from the heart, carbon dioxide is passed from the blood through the alveolar wall, to the air, and oxygen is passed from the air, through the alveolar wall, to the blood. There it can be taken to the heart and then pumped to the rest of the body. When the alveolar walls rupture they cannot function properly, and result in the condition called emphysema, or heaves.

What makes this marvelous course of events take place? The lungs sit within the thorax in a vacuum system. A very thin sheet of tissue, called *pleura*, lines the inside of the thorax and also lines the outside of the lungs. The pleura is kept slightly moist by the body and the moisture serves to hold a vacuum between the two pleural-covered structures, much like denture adhesive forms a bond to hold dentures to the gums. (Pleurisy is a condition of friction when adequate moisture is lacking between the two layers.) If the internal size of the thorax increases the size of the lungs must also increase, and there is only one way for that to occur—by air entering through the trachea. Conversely, as thoracic size decreases so must the size of the lungs, a process known as exhalation.

Although there are many muscles responsible for regulating the size of the chest cavity the most important has to be the *diaphragm*. Forming the boundary between the thorax and abdomen, the diaphragm actually consists of three muscles and a very broad thin tendon. At the top are two small muscles, a *left and right crus*. These surround the *aorta* as it carries blood from the thorax to the structures in the back of the body. The right crus, the larger of the two cura, also has a hole in it through which passes the *esophagus* on its way to the stomach. Attached to the ribs and sternum, completing the circle formed by the cura, is the *muscular skirt* with its centrally oriented muscle fibers. The space in the center of the diaphragm not occupied

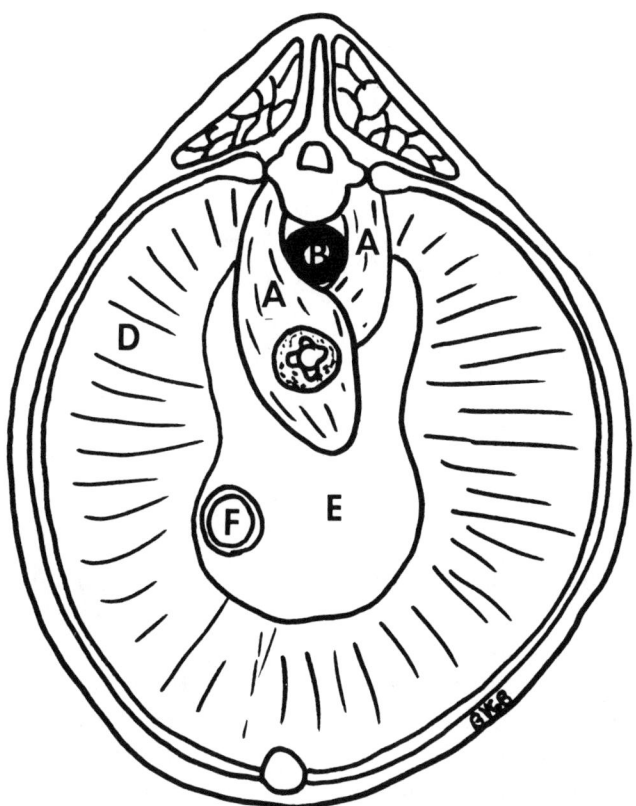

FIGURE 21. **The Diaphragm: A–Right and Left Cura; B–Aorta; C–Esophagus; D–Muscular Skirt; E–Central Tendon; F–Caudal Vena Cava.**

by muscle is the *central tendon* and through its opening passes the *caudal vena cava* returning blood from the abdomen to the heart. Two nerves, the left and right *phrenic nerves*, course through the thorax between the two lungs to supply the diaphragm, directing it when to contract. This direction results in the shortening of muscle fibers, pulling abdominal structures back and increasing space within the thoracic cavity, causing inspiration.

5
A Ticker at Work (The Circulatory System)

The beating of the heart is the result of one small organ pumping blood throughout the body. The heart, then, is more than a symbol of Valentine's Day, it is a symbol of life.

Venous blood is used blood returning to be reoxygeninated, detoxified, and repumped to the body. At the heart, this blood enters from two main routes. The *cranial vena cava* returns blood from the head and thoracic limb, while most veins from structures behind the heart merge into the *caudal vena cava*. Both of these large veins open into a thin walled chamber, the *right atrium*. Here blood is held until the next chamber has been emptied. The right atrium has an *auricle*, a flap-like appendage, to help increase the storage capacity of the chamber.

In natural progression, blood will pass through the *right atrioventricular (A-V) valve* into the *right ventricle*. This lower chamber has a muscular wall because its primary function is to pump the blood out. Several other features are unique to the ventricle, including muscular columns with thin cords attaching to the parts of the right A-V valve. This arrangement of muscle and cords is highly desirable because as the chamber contracts to push blood out, these structures prevent the right A-V valve from opening up into the right atrium. This allows the right A-V valve to be a one-way valve with blood flowing only from atrium to ventricle, never the reverse.

As blood leaves the right ventricle it passes a second valve, the *pulmonary valve*. Although shaped differently than the A-V valve the pulmonary valve also is one-way, allowing blood to flow out of the heart into the *pulmonary arteries*. These arteries carry the blood to the lungs where some waste products are removed and oxygen is added.

Once purified, the blood is returned to the *left atrium* by way of the *pulmonary veins*. The left atrium is somewhat smaller than its right counterpart, but it looks and functions are the same.

Blood now flows past the *left atrioventricular* (A-V) *valve*, another one-way safeguard, into the *left ventricle*. Although the internal structure of this chamber is much the same as that of the right ventricle, the muscular wall is several times thicker. The pumping action of the left ventricle must push blood throughout all the vessels of the body, whereas that of the right ventricle need only push blood to the lungs and back, and the muscular effort is therefore considerably different. Thus the difference in size of the ventricles.

To leave the heart the blood passes the last of the four valves, the *aortic valve*, and enters the main artery of the body, the *aorta*. From this vessel it is distributed to all tissues of the body. Very near the origin of the aorta, two *coronary arteries* leave to furnish blood directly to the muscle of the heart itself. It is an acute blockage of one of these coronary arteries that results in a heart attack, rare in the horse but common in man. The next important structure requiring blood is the brain, and the next artery branching from the aorta therefore supplies the head.

If during the trip through the heart the blood encounters something that disrupts the normal flow, such as a hole between chambers or a valve that won't close, a heart murmur results. A murmur is the sound resulting from turbulent blood flow, while the "lub-dub" of the normal heart beat is the sound of the valves closing.

As blood flows through the body it progresses into arteries of decreasing size. At the smallest size, a vessel called a *capillary*, the actual exchange of oxygen and waste products occurs. Something else happens at this level. Blood is composed of two portions, the cells (red and white blood cells) and liquid (serum). At the capillary level the cells pass through one at a time along with a small amount of serum. The rest of the fluid leaves the capillaries and travels through the tissue. At the end of the capillary most of the fluid reenters the vessel and travels through the veins back to the heart. Some fluid does not go back into the blood stream. Now called *lymph*, this fluid is picked up by lymphatic vessels which end by carrying their contents to the cranial vena cava. Enroute the lymph may be occasionally filtered by passing through structures called *lymph nodes*. If harmful bacteria or cancer cells are picked up by the lymph, they may be stopped from spreading to the rest of the body by a lymph node.

6
Eat, Drink, and Be Sick (The Digestive System)

Food usually enters the mouth, having been gathered by the front teeth and lips. These front incisors have a flat sharp surface to help tear grass loose from its roots. The tongue helps move the grass or grain to the back of the mouth where it is ground into finer pieces and mixed with saliva. Improper growth or wear on teeth produces a number of conditions resulting in a decreased ability to grind and thus digest available food.

Young horses shed their *deciduous* ("baby") *teeth* just like people do. The root is partially dissolved to loosen it, before the tooth is lost, and the new tooth pushes the old one out. The deciduous cheek teeth of the horse tend to hollow out inside as the root dissolves. As the new tooth pushes up it may become wedged inside the baby tooth, which then has trouble being shed. The remaining baby tooth, called a cap, causes difficulty in chewing and must be removed.

The coming, going, and wear of teeth provide a method of determining the age of the animal. There are certain principles which should be mentioned for a general understanding of aging a horse by its teeth. The most accurate method of age determination is to identify when upper and lower incisors fall out or come in. These ages are consistant to within six or eight months. The upper and lower central four deciduous teeth (central incisors) are shed between 2½ and 3 years of age. The teeth next to each of the centrals (intermediate incisors) are lost between 3½ and 4 years of age. The corner incisors are shed at about age 4½ to 5 years, and in each case the new permanent tooth should appear shortly thereafter. Determining age by wear on the lower incisors is the second most accurate form, and this becomes highly variable with increased age and with the consumption of large amounts of dirt or sand. A horse's teeth are constantly growing, in contrast to those of most other animals which have only a short growth period. This causes them to change shape and results in changes in the identifiable parts of the teeth. Diets which cause excessive wear to the teeth can result in a "tooth age" of several years older than the animal's true age.

The roof of the horse's mouth consists of two areas, the *hard palate*, with its tissue covering boney ridges, and the *soft palate*, a continuation of the soft tissue behind the end of the bone. Both palates function to keep the air and food passages separate. The soft palate of the horse is extremely long in comparison to that of other animals, and because of this the horse cannot mouth-breathe. The weight and length of the structure cover up the opening at the back of the mouth, and air must enter the *trachea* ("windpipe") from the nose. This is also the reason that stomach tubes must go through the nose of the horse rather than the mouth. Tubes usually are not strong enough to lift the weight of the soft palate without injuring it. Muscles elevate this structure during swallowing, while a special piece of cartilage, the *epiglottis*, blocks the opening of the trachea to allow food to pass.

As food is swallowed it enters the *esophagus* ("food tube"), inside which it passes down the neck. The esophagus is usually above the trachea, except in the middle of the neck where it is above and to the left of the trachea. Visualization of a stomach tube passing through the esophagus can occur at this location. This observation assures that materials go to the stomach and not the lungs. As the esophagus passes through the *thorax* ("chest") it is again above the trachea, and then passes through a special hole in the diaphragm.

Once within the abdomen the esophagus soon opens into the *stomach*, the large storage area. The horse has a stomach which is shaped and functions much like the human stomach. If the digestive system functions continuously, it is obvious that food must then be continuously supplied. This is the job of the stomach, to store food which enters at peak eating periods and then release it slowly during the entire day.

The *small intestine* is the next pathway along the line of travel, and is the location for digestion of everything except grass and hay. Special ducts carrying digestive enzymes from the *liver* and *pancreas* open into the first few feet of this lengthy area. These glandular enzymes break food down into simpler forms which can be absorbed through the intestinal wall. The absorbed products are then picked up by the bloodstream and carried to the liver for storage or distribution. After winding through most of the abdomen in the small intestine whatever food remaining enters the *large intestine*. The *cecum* is a large pouch at the start of the large intestine, and is functionally important in the horse. (Humans have a small, nonfunctional cecum which happens to have a second small nonfunctional pouch attached to it, the appendix.) Food enters the top of the cecum and is mixed through this organ. It is here that special organisms break down the grasses so that these too can serve a nutritional function. (Grasses eaten by cattle, sheep, and goats are broken down in special compartments of the stomach which the horse does not have.)

After being processed in the cecum the food again comes to the top and enters the *colon*, which is uniquely designed in the horse. The first portion is very elongated as compared to that in the human, and in addition is very wide. Forming a large double "U", it reaches from the right abdominal floor, to the front of the abdomen, along the left side, folds on itself, and reverses direction back to the right side. Occasionally these areas of large intestine twist on themselves, stopping the blood supply to the area and resulting in colic.

Food passes from the dilated portion of the large intestine into the much smaller terminal sections. Occasionally this process does not occur easily, causing pain and sometimes even blockage and colic. Water is removed in the last portions of the colon to give fecal matter the consistency we are accustomed to shoveling after it has passed from the colon to the *rectum* and through the *anus*.

Although the horse can be infested with several different types of parasites, the large strongyles are definitely the most destructive. These comprise one type of what are commonly called bloodworms. Most large strongyles, which belong to the genus *Strongylus*, live by attaching to the tissue which lines the colon. This will damage the lining of the colon and can result in digestive problems, but something much worse than that can happen. *Strongylus vulgaris* is the most destructive member of this group of parasites, damaging the arteries in over ninety percent of all horses! Blood vessels are lined with a membrane called the *tunica intima* ("internal coat"), which keeps blood cells from sticking to the vessel and forming a clot. For reasons not fully understood, *S. vulgaris* gets into the arteries, usually the major artery to the intestines (the *cranial mesenteric artery*), and by doing so injures the tunica intima of the vessel where it enters. This injury, located at the start of the artery, causes the vessel to become greatly thickened and the intima to become crumbly and flaky. Pieces of this damaged lining can break off and travel farther down the blood vessel until the vessel narrows and the intima piece plugs the small artery. This sometimes temporarily interferes with the blood supply to the intestines, resulting in one form of colic.

Small strongyles are another grouping of internal equine parasites which also live in the colon. These are also commonly called bloodworms.

Oxyuris equi is a common intestinal parasite in horses. Its more common name is pinworm, but it is NOT related to human pinworms. This parasite doesn't cause much internal damage to the horse but can cause itching in the anal area, often resulting in tail rubbing.

Roundworms, or ascarids *(Parascaris equorum)*, are often seen by the horse owner in the horse's droppings. These worms are much more frequent in young horses, probably because with age an immunity, a kind of a self-vaccination develops against them. Attachment to the small intestine can cause some damage to this organ, and occasionally a hole all the way through the intestine can be created.

Strongyloides are other parasites of young foals and have caused severe diarrhea. Again, immunity develops to some extent with age.

During the summer, bot flies become a real problem. The fly is the adult form of the *Gasterophilus species* and the eggs they lay are deposited in areas where the horse can get them into its mouth. The immature larval forms of this fly attach to the lining of the stomach and can do considerable damage to it.

Even horses can have tapeworms, and like pinworms, they do not infest the human. Little damage is usually done to the intestinal track, but ulcers can occur near the junction of the small and large intestines, a very important area in the horse.

Control of internal parasites in the horse is accomplished in several ways, one of which is worming. With several different types of internal parasites, each may require a different type of worming medicine to be killed. The only sure way to know the kinds of parasites that are living inside the horse is to do a fecal examination, looking under a microscope for the eggs of the various parasites. Only then can the appropriate medication be selected.

The method of treatment can vary from medicine put in the feed to medicine administered through a stomach tube. This last method is probably best because the horse gets entire dose of wormer without either picking out individual granules or not eating all his feed at one time. Each of us is probably familiar with the horse that can eat his feed while picking out every worming granule mixed with it. One type of wormer added to feed is made of dichlorvos. This active ingredient is a vapor attached to a pellet or granule. The vapor is released within the digestive track, so don't be surprised to see the granules looking unchanged when they are in the feces. This is the same chemical used in the hanging insect strips and in flea collars.

During the next trip to the feed store, look at the packages of various worming medications. Most claim they kill several kinds of parasites. What they don't say is that they may kill ninety-five percent of one type of worm but only 10 percent to 25 percent of the others, depending on the medicine. The 95 percent type may be a type of worm your horse doesn't even have—wasted money. The best way to know if a particular wormer is adequate is to ask your veterinarian about its ingredients or to have him or her worm the horse for you. All worming medications are poisons and are made to be more poisonous to the parasite than to the horse. This is the main reason it is important to give the horse only the amount of wormer the directions call for. Don't give the little "extra"—it could mean a sick or dead horse.

Is one worm-control program best? The best program is a routine one based on your geographic location. Horses in the southern states should be wormed every two to three months. In the northern states three times a year may be adequate if done in early spring, summer, and late fall, after a killing frost. The immature forms of internal parasites are passed in the feces and must be eaten to infest the horse. Freezing will kill them, as will heating and drying. The latter can be accomplished by spreading manure where horses can't get it until it has dried. Fly control and removal of bot fly eggs certainly are indicated in a good control program. A parasite-free horse is a healthy horse and a healthy horse both looks and feels better.

Probably the most dreaded word in a horseman's vocabulary is "colic." It is also one of those veterinarians hate to hear. Colic refers to the signs shown by a horse with abdominal pain. Because horses have a low tolerance of pain, they show signs of pain in situations that wouldn't bother humans, cows, or dogs. Something like "acid indigestion" to us results in a lot of complaining while we take our Tums or Rolaids, but a similiar pain in the horse could be seen as colic. (By the way, horses can't burp or vomit so gas pressure can build up in them.)

Normal behavior patterns change and the affected animal is very restless, lying down and getting up repeatedly. Usually it tries to roll. Occasionally it may lie in the corner of its stall with its feet in the air. Grunting and groaning are common, and the horse may look at its side or even kick or nip at it. Sweating is also common, and usually the horse has a tense anxious look on its face.

What causes colic signs? The list would be endless. Often in treating colic the veterinarian treats the most probable cause, hoping the condition isn't resulting from something really serious. During the winter, especially in northern states, horses tend to drink less water than they should because the water is so cold, and in the hot southern summers the animal will sweat off a lot of its water. The food moving through the intestines therefore has less water to make it slippery and is harder to move. This is called a partial impaction, and is treated with mineral oil by stomach tube to help lubricate the dry food mass and by other drugs to help ease the pain. Overstretching of intestines by a large passage of food causing pain would also be treated the same way.

Twists in the intestine can cause colic, and we are probably all familiar with someone who has had the misfortune of losing a horse from a twisted intestine. In this condition the twist stops the supply of blood to a part of the intestine, which will then die. What happens to a piece of meat left outside on a warm day? The same is happening inside this horse. The "dead meat," or intestine, is inside a warm wrapper (the abdominal cavity) and is starting to rot. The breakdown products or toxins are being picked up and distributed throughout the body while the pain from the twist causes the horse to show signs of colic. Obviously, surgery would be the most successful method of treatment.

In the horse the *Strongylus vulgaris* causes damage to the main artery to the intestines. Pieces of this enlarged damaged artery can break off and travel down arterial branches until it reaches one smaller than itself. This causes a temporary loss of blood to a small piece of intestine, another painful situation to the horse. He reacts by showing signs of colic.

Infections within the abdominal cavity can also be painful. Mares in foal may show some colic from temporary pressure on one of the arteries. These are just a very few of the problems that can cause colic. Fortunately, partial impactions are the most common cause and most horses respond well to treatment.

The usual advice someone gets for dealing with a horse with colic is to keep that animal moving. Why should we force an animal in pain to walk? The usual cause of this condition is a partial intestinal obstruction, and this is relatively easy to treat. If the horse can get down and roll, it can also twist part of the intestine, resulting in an even worse problem that is extremely difficult to diagnose and treat.

7
A Waste Disposal Plant (The Urinary System)

Of all the organs of a horse's body, four are essential. The heart must beat to pump over ten gallons of blood throughout the body. Without the oxygen exchange in the lungs breath is impossible, and so is life. Central control of all body functions, including the circulatory and respiratory systems, is absolutely essential, and so the brain is needed. The fourth organ which must function is the *kidney*. This paired-filter system is nature's method of eliminating wastes from the blood.

Each horse is born with two kidneys, located under the last few ribs to the right or left of the vertebral column. In this position they are well protected from outside injuries. A layer of fat surrounding them also protects by serving as a cushion against bruises and bumps. The surface of these organs is relatively smooth in the horse, as opposed to lobated (lumpy) in cattle. Also lacking is the typical "bean" shape as seen in most other animals.

Gross observation of the kidney shows several prominent features. Closely attached to the outside is a "skin-like" coat, the *renal capsule*. This helps prevent swelling of the kidney, enabling it to function more efficiently. The kidney tissue itself can be divided visually into an outer layer, the *cortex* and an inner layer, the *medulla*. These areas represent different portions of the functioning units. Near the center is a hollow space, the *renal sinus*, which contains fat, an artery, a vein, and a funnel-like structure, the *renal pelvis*.

Within the cortex and medulla of each kidney are hundreds of thousands of microscopic filtration units called *nephrons* and it is in these units that blood purification occurs. Two large arteries leave the aorta (primary artery of the body), one going to each kidney. As these *renal arteries* enter their respective kidneys, they divide into smaller and smaller branches. Eventually each branch curls into a little "tuft" called a *glomerulus*, and it soon straightens out again. *Bowman's capsule* is the "C" shaped end of each nephron which encircles the glomerulus to receive the fluid leaving the glomerular artery. Blood cells are relatively large and cannot escape from the vessel, but the fluid can.

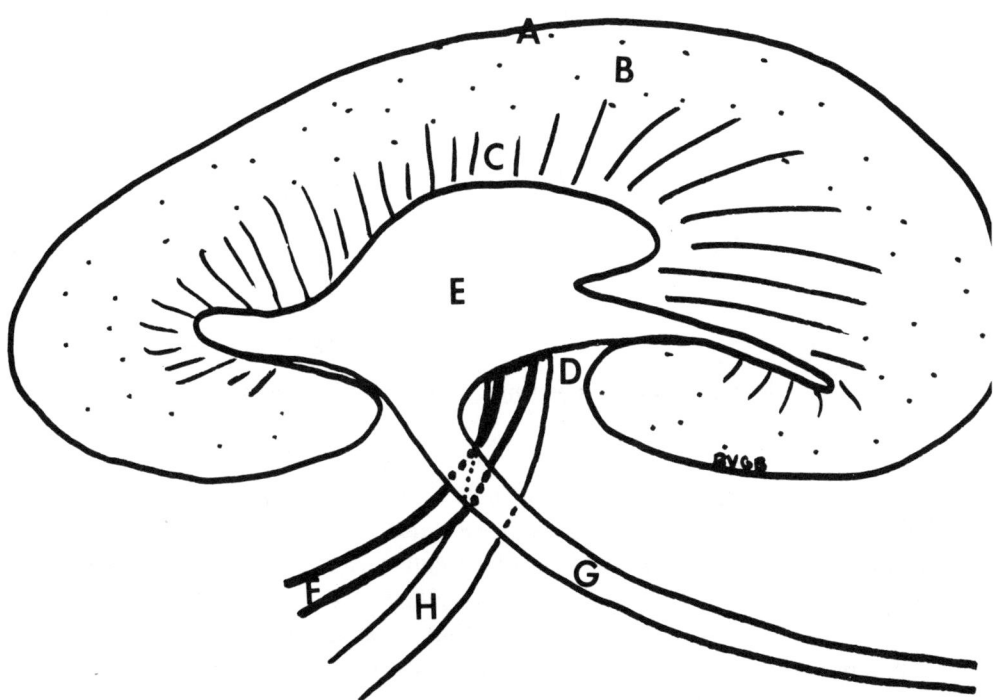

FIGURE 22. The Kidney: A–Renal Capsule; B–Renal Cortex; C–Renal Medulla; D–Renal Sinus; E–Renal Pelvis; F–Renal Artery; G–Ureter; H–Renal Vein.

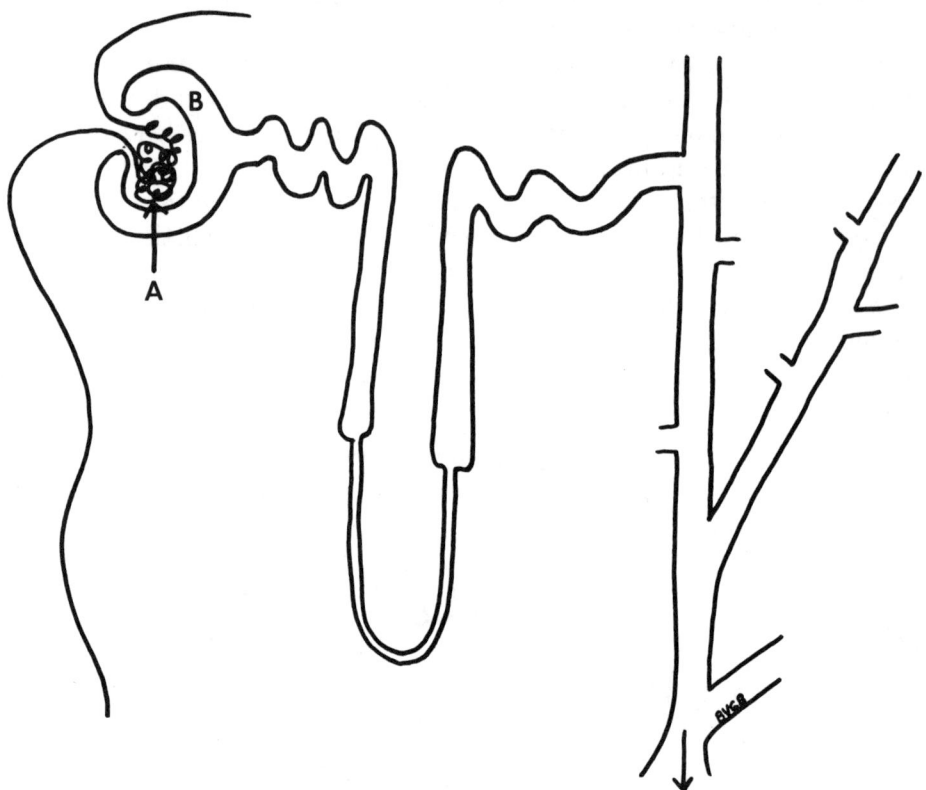

FIGURE 23. **A Nephron: A–Glomerulus; B–Bowman's Capsule.**

   Once inside the nephron, the fluid passes through the tubular passageways, and here the purification process is really at work. Because of pressure differences between fluids on the inside and outside of the tubules, and because of concentration differences of such things as sodium, sugar, and nitrogen between the fluids inside and outside of the tubules, fluids and the other substances can be actively moved out or can remain inside the nephron. As the fluid reaches the end of the nephron the excess substances are kept in the urine while the amount of fluid needed by the body has been drawn out. The result is urine, which is then collected from all the nephrons of each kidney. The collection area, the renal pelvis, serves much like the wide part of a funnel, bringing the urine flow into the *ureter*. Most of the fluid which enters Bowman's capsule is reabsorbed by the body, leaving the tubules and entering the small veins which surround them. These is a hollow space, the *renal sinus,* which contains fat, an artery, a vein, and a funnel-like structure, the *renal pelvis.*

Within the cortex and medulla of each kidney are hundreds of thousands of microscopic filtration units called *nephrons* and it is in these units that blood purification occurs. Two large arteries leave the aorta (primary artery of the body), one going to each kidney. As these *renal arteries* enter their respective kidneys, they divide into smaller and smaller branches. Eventually each branch curls into a little "tuft" called a *glomerulus,* and it soon straightens out again. *Bowman's capsule* is the "C" shaped end of each nephron which encircles the glomerulus to receive the fluid leaving the glomerular artery. Blood cells are relatively large and cannot escape from the vessel, but the fluid can.

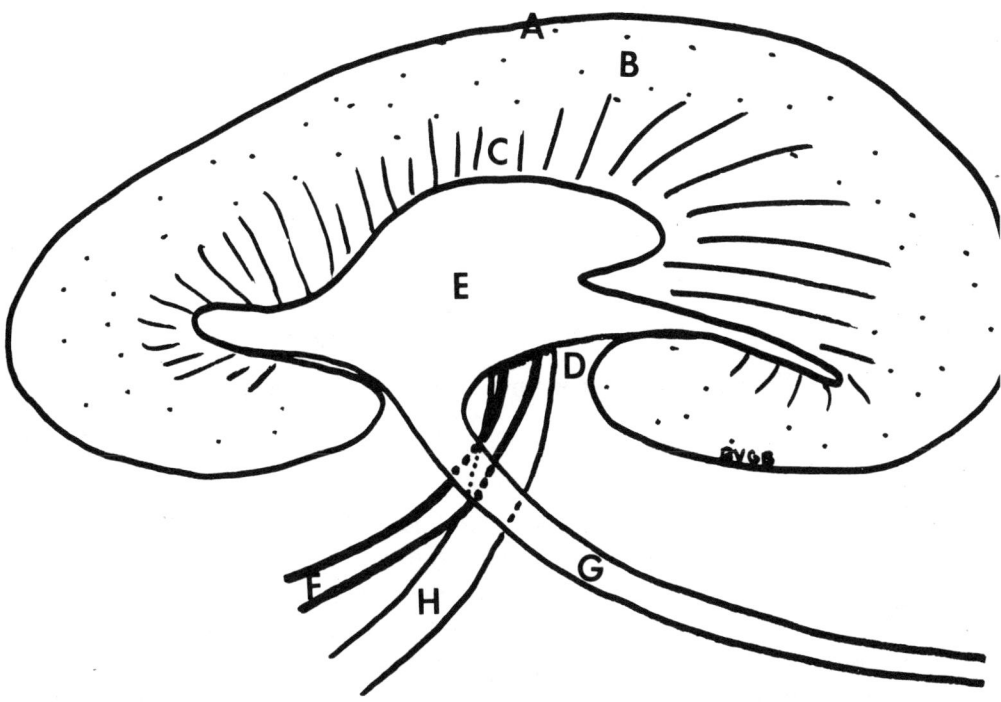

FIGURE 22. The Kidney: A–Renal Capsule; B–Renal Cortex; C–Renal Medulla; D–Renal Sinus; E–Renal Pelvis; F–Renal Artery; G–Ureter; H–Renal Vein.

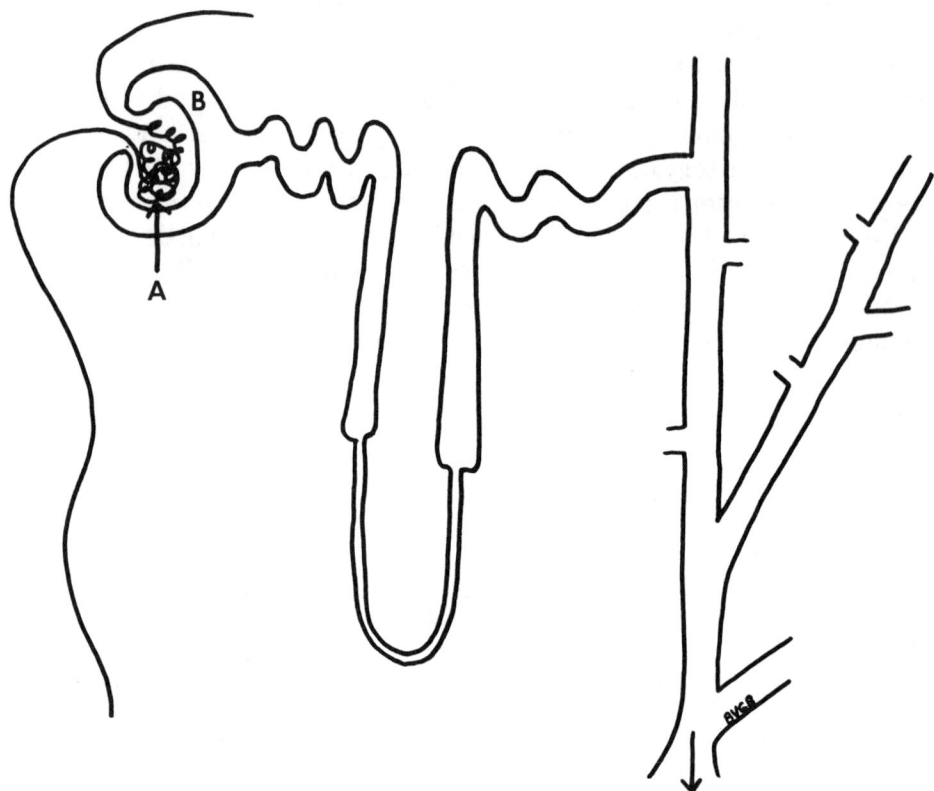

FIGURE 23. **A Nephron: A–Glomerulus; B–Bowman's Capsule.**

Once inside the nephron, the fluid passes through the tubular passageways, and here the purification process is really at work. Because of pressure differences between fluids on the inside and outside of the tubules, and because of concentration differences of such things as sodium, sugar, and nitrogen between the fluids inside and outside of the tubules, fluids and the other substances can be actively moved out or can remain inside the nephron. As the fluid reaches the end of the nephron the excess substances are kept in the urine while the amount of fluid needed by the body has been drawn out. The result is urine, which is then collected from all the nephrons of each kidney. The collection area, the renal pelvis, serves much like the wide part of a funnel, bringing the urine flow into the *ureter*. Most of the fluid which enters Bowman's capsule is reabsorbed by the body, leaving the tubules and entering the small veins which surround them. These veins will join to each other so that one renal vein carries all blood from the kidney to the caudal vena cava.

Each of the two ureters connects a kidney to the *urinary bladder*, located within the abdomen just ahead of the pelvis. Here it is stored until the horse determines it is time to urinate, usually just after entering a newly bedded stall.

A real safety factor has been built into the kidney to protect the body from its loss. As much as three-fourths of the total kidney function in some animals can be lost before waste products build up in the blood. And even then, the build-up is at a slow rate.

Azoturia is an old problem from the draft horse era that is on the increase again. You may have heard of it as Monday Morning Disease, Sore Kidneys, or Tied-up, and it is very similiar to White Muscle Disease in cattle. Draft horses were worked hard during the week and rested on Saturday and Sunday, while often being kept on full working feed seven days a week. When the animal was worked hard again on Monday, the condition showed up. Today we see show horses fed a lot of grain to keep them fat who then become sick when worked relatively hard on the weekend during a show (kind of an early "Monday").

Signs that we see with azoturia usually show up first in the rear legs. The horse "moves funny," not lame, but stiff. Usually the animal becomes more reluctant to move and the hind leg muscles feel hard. Also seen is an increase in body temperature, which is an indication of the pain the horse is in. In extreme cases the horse can literally drop in its tracks. The *loin* area (along the back, just ahead of the hips) is sensitive to pressure. A touch there usually causes the horse to "sink down." If urination occurs, the urine color is usually a very dark yellow-brown.

Why do we see these signs? Horses fed high grain rations are getting a lot of protein, which is stored in the muscles. Hard work causes the body to break down muscle protein, leaving it as a waste product in the blood. A small amount of this waste product is of no bother to the horse but in excessive amounts, as results from hard work, can cause severe damage to the kidneys. It's like trying to push big sticks through small holes. The damaged kidneys are painful (pain over the loin), they back up waste products into the blood (seen as rear leg stiffness), and pass abnormal materials, like the protein wastes, into the urine (dark urine).

What first-aid measures should be taken until a veterinarian arrives? First of all, stop working that horse. Get off it, remove the saddle, and give it rest. Don't feed it anything, especially grain, but do see that it gets plenty of water. (Remember that if you have been working it very hard, only offer small amounts of water until the animal has cooled off. It wouldn't be good to compound azoturia with founder.) This is not a condition to take lightly. A horse could die from it.

In azoturia the kidneys have been damaged and need time to repair. Once affected, diet and exercise will have to be properly controlled so that azoturia doesn't reoccur.

8
Foals Don't Come from Eggs (The Genital System)

In order to understand the entire reproductive process in the mare it is necessary to understand something about mare's anatomy. Basic reproductive anatomy is similiar in all females regardless of species, although individual parts may vary in size.

Eggs are produced in the *ovary* which is located near the back of the abdominal cavity. In the horse the ovaries are approximately the size of a small lemon and will change shape somewhat as the mare nears her *estrous* ("heat") period. During that time, watery cyst-like structures appear, the location of maturing eggs. When the egg is released during heat it becomes free of the ovary at an indented area on the surface of the ovary called the *ovulation fossa*. The *oviduct* ("fallopian tube", "salpinx", "uterine tube") is a small tube which carries the egg to the uterus, and it is in the oviduct where fertilization of the egg by male sperm must take place for pregnancy to occur. The part of the oviduct nearest to the ovary, the *infundibulum*, is flared out to collect the egg, and causes the entire structure to resemble a funnel.

It takes the egg a few days to pass through the oviduct and enter the *uterus*. The mare's uterus is shaped like a "T" with the base called the *body of the uterus* and the left and right crosspieces called the *uterine horns*. The uterus is where the fertilized egg will stay and develop during pregnancy. This is the structure your veterinarian is feeling for when palpating a mare to see if she is pregnant.

66 • Your Horse's Health

The *cervix* is a structure located at the far end of the body of the uterus which functions to open and close the uterus to the outside. While in heat the mare has a relaxed cervix, allowing sperm to enter the uterus, but when not in heat the cervix is closed so as to keep *bacteria* ("germs") from getting in. During pregnancy the cervix is more tightly closed by a plug of mucus, preventing the foal and its membranes from being expelled.

Past the cervix is an area called the *vagina*. Many mares develop an infection here, and it becomes difficult to settle them. Bacteria will often kill the stallion's sperm and conception cannot occur. Back of the vagina is the *vestibule*, a region that is shared by both the urinary system and the reproductive system. The vestibule opens to the

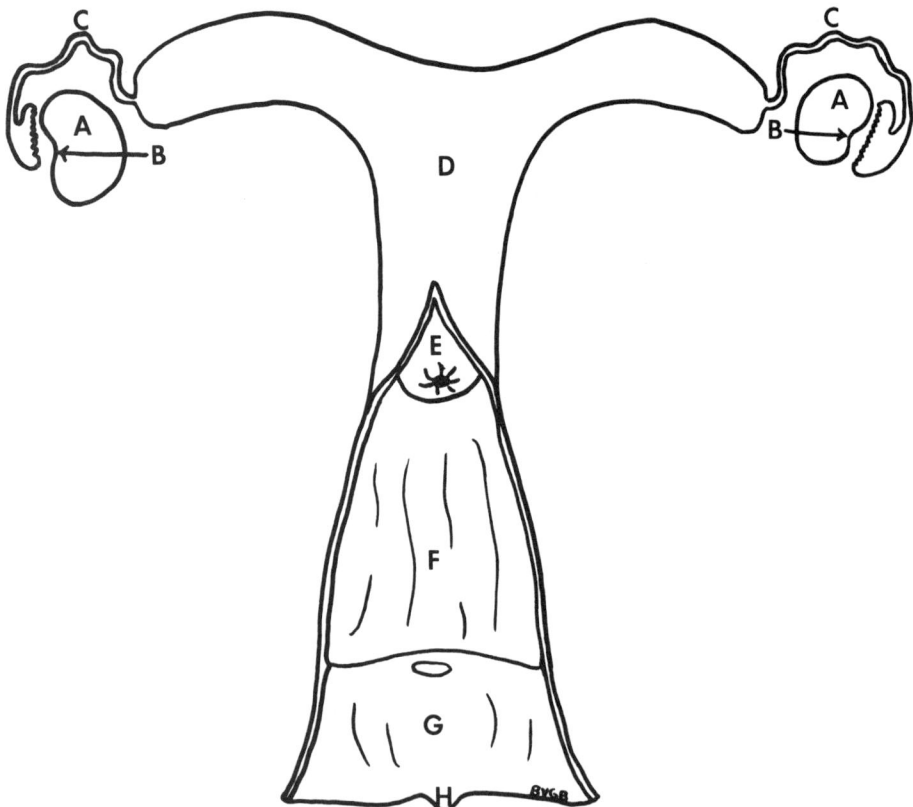

FIGURE 24. **Female Reproductive Tract, Top View: A–Ovary; B–Ovulation Fossa; C–Oviduct; D–Uterus; E–Cervix; F–Vagina; G–Vestibule; H–Vulva.**

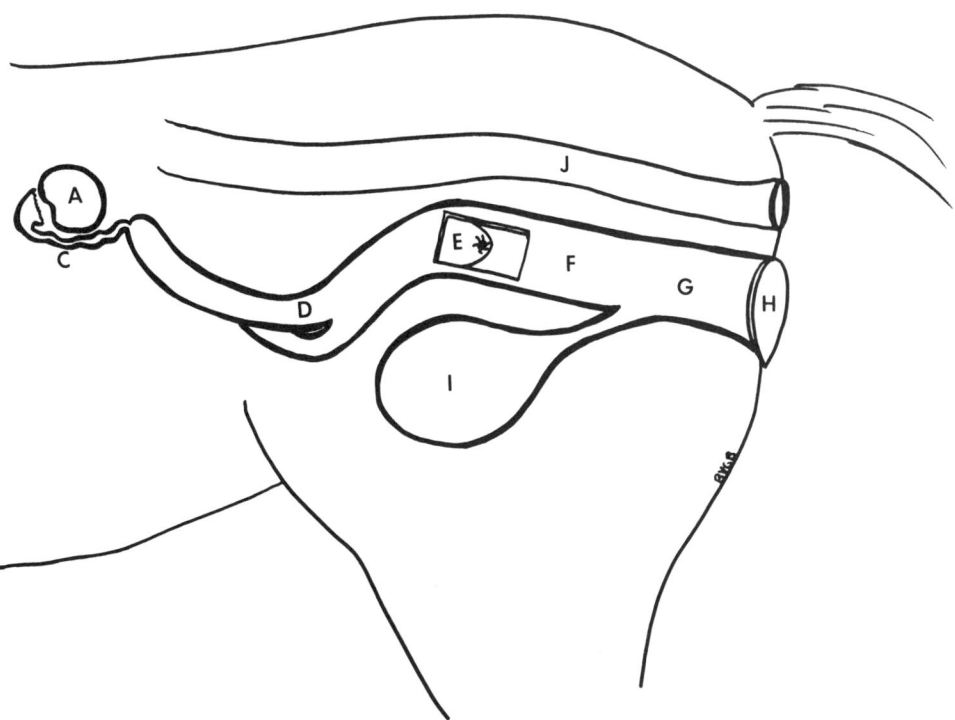

FIGURE 25. **Female Reproductive Tract, Side View: A–Ovary; C–Oviduct; D–Uterus; E–Cervix; F–Vagina; G–Vestibule; H–Vulva; I–Urinary Bladder; J–Rectum.**

outside of the mare at the *vulva*. The vagina, vestibule, and vulva together are called the *birth canal*. This will stretch to a considerable extent during foaling, limited mainly by the size of the mare's pelvis. This is the primary reason it is so important to look for a good width in the hip of a mare's conformation.

In addition to understanding the normal anatomy of the mare's reproductive tract, it is also desirable to learn about accompanying normal physiology and behavior. Usually called the heat cycle, the estrous cycle in a mare is a very complex series of events which is reflected externally as changes in behavior.

A mare generally has a heat cycle every nineteen to twenty-three days (twenty-one days is average), and the outward signs of heat show for two to nine days (five is average), although this is somewhat longer in draft breed mares. It is during this two-to nine-day period that the mare will accept the stallion, and often her personality is somewhat different than at other times. Individual mares may vary from this pattern but the majority will follow it quite closely. These nineteen-to twenty-three-day cycles repeat themselves during the year to form one of three types of breeding cycles.

A monoestrous breeding cycle most frequently occurs in the wild horse breeds. It usually has four or five estrous cycles and occurs during the longest days of the year. The mare with this type of cycle is only capable of becoming pregnant during approximately four months of the year, usually May to August.

As transitory polyoestrus, a mare has estrous cycles during almost the entire year. This means she will come in heat every nineteen to twenty-three days throughout the year. The tricky part about this type of breeding cycle is that an egg is released by her ovary only during the early part of the year (December to August, depending on the location in the country). This means she can be bred in September or November but would not become pregnant because no egg had been released. Mares in the southern part of the United States have been shown to have fertile heats earlier in the year than those in the northern part due to light differences. Stud farms are now offering controlled lighting to bring mares into fertile heat periods sooner.

True polyoestrous breeding cycles occur in mares that have heat cycles and ovulate throughout the year, and are therefore capable of becoming pregnant during any one of their heat periods. With the tendency for early foals, this type of cycle is favored in many breeding programs.

Mares come into heat more gradually than do most other domestic animals. When not in heat, mares are very defensive against a stallion which shows interest. This animosity decreases as heat approaches so that a mare will tolerate a stallion smelling and nipping at her. Owners will notice that the mare urinates more often, but in smaller amounts. When in full heat most mares will indicate readiness to breed in several ways when a stallion is near. She will stand with hind legs spread apart, her tail is held to one side, and after urinating the vulva edges are opened and closed several times in rapid succession.

Changes in the mare's behavior can include personality changes. Often we wish something could be done to prevent these changes. Although some mares show almost no behavorial differences when they cycle, other mares show extreme changes to the point of kicking, biting, or bucking. Owners are unhappy about their decreased chances for success in the show ring and have resorted to other options.

There are three courses of action which can be taken by mare owners. First on the list is learning to tolerate the cycling mare, leaving her at home if necessary during her heat period. Mares which are always in heat should be checked by a veterinarian because ovarian cysts or tumors can cause these signs. Advantages for accepting this natural cycle include the fact you will have a breedable mare when her show career ends. Disadvantages include inconvenience to you, as mares seem to delight at coming in heat during large important shows. The selection process used by nature to develop the modern horse obviously favors mares showing strong estrous periods to those hardly showing estrous behavior, because these were more easily identified by the stallion. Modern man is reversing this selection process for his convenience.

A second method to handle mares which are problems during the estrous cycle is to spay them. The ovaries can be surgically removed, the operation usually done with the horse standing and not involving the general anesthesia as is used to spay a dog. (To contrast the surgeries: in women the uterus is usually removed, a hysterectomy; in dogs and cats the ovaries and the uterus are removed, an ovariohysterectomy; in horses the ovaries are removed, an ovariotomy.) With no ovaries present, the mare will not have a heat cycle and thus will not exhibit the associated behavior changes. The obvious disadvantage is that the mare will not be able to produce a foal, but examine that disadvantage in another light. Approximately 50 percent of all foals are stallions, and the majority of these are neutered because their behavior is undesirable and because their conformation is less than ideal. The other 50 percent of the foals are mares, so why shouldn't they be neutered because their behavior is undesirable or because their conformation is less than ideal? Behavior is an inherited trait, just as conformation is. To prevent the possibility of buying a spayed mare as a future brood mare insist on a prepurchase physical examination, including a genital exam, conducted by your veterinarian. This will also protect you against such things as blindness and unsoundness in the mare you purchase. Spayed mares have a very definite place in the horse world, as do geldings.

A third method is used to handle estrous cycle problems in mares—hormones. These have been used to take mares out of heat and to bring mares into heat, but their complications *greatly* outweigh their advantages in both cases. The results are unpredictable at best and often produce more problems than they solve. Did you ever wonder why some of the best show mares continued to be shown for years past their prime and then retired never to be heard from again? Some of these were treated with hormones, became sterile, and couldn't produce foals. Some were then given hormones to bring them into heat, but that type of heat usually doesn't have a mature egg to be fertilized. Natural body hormones are produced in amounts so small that very complicated procedures are needed to even measure them. Then man interfers with an injection thousands of times more potent than the normal amounts, usually given during the wrong part of the cycle, and then he wonders why the entire hormone system is thrown out of whack! Only in a few clinical cases can hormone therapy be justified.

There can be several reasons why a mare won't settle into a normal pregnancy. Some of these reasons are easy to correct, some are not, but each must be corrected, if possible, before a foal can be produced.

The human element in a breeding operation is responsible for at least half the problems in not settling mares. Obviously, the future mother must be in good physical condition in order to settle. This means she is neither starving nor fat. With former show horses fat is a real and significant problem, not only to normal conception but also to uncomplicated foaling and foal health if the mare does become pregnant. In most modern breeding operations, a mare is "hand bred," meaning that the stallion is brought to the mare and mating occurs while the stallion is still controlled by a halter and lead. Pasture breeding is occasionally used on larger ranches that don't breed outside mares. Hand breeding introduces another human element—humans decide when in the cycle to breed that mare, and that decision is often based on a calendar rather than on what the mare's ovary is doing.

A mare can be responsible for not settling. Some mares exhibit a "silent heat," which means they are inwardly cycling but don't exhibit outward behavorial signs of an estrous mare. Hormone levels could also be off, producing a mare with irregular or no estrous cycles. Ovarian tumors and cysts are just two causes fitting into this heading, but these are not extremely common.

Infections are common reasons for mares not settling. These infections of the vagina or the uterus can result in a mare that no longer cycles or in one that cycles but doesn't conceive because the sperm are killed by the infection. Many stallion owners require that outside mares be cultured by a veterinarian to check for the presence of infection before breeding season. This serves two purposes. First it prevents an infected mare from infecting the stallion, and thus prevents him from infecting other mares. Secondly it gives the mare every possible chance to settle, decreasing the number of repeat breedings.

Windsucker conformation helps to bring infectious agents inside the mare. In this type of conformation, the anus looks like it has sunken into the mare. This causes the vulva to be drawn both higher than normal and farther back than the anus. When the horse eliminates feces, the fecal matter will fall on the vulva and bacteria in the feces can easily be drawn into the vestibule and uterus. When urinating, the mare's urine would also have to flow uphill through the vestibule if the conformation were that of a windsucker. Instead some of it flows forward, irritating the vagina wall and making it more susceptible to infections when bacteria get in. A Caslick's operation is one where the edges of the vulva are sutured shut to help stop bacteria from getting in. In racing mares the edges of the vulva will sometimes flap open and shut, producing pain and resulting in the mare not wanting to run. For this reason a Caslick's operation is routinely done on all mares going into race training, not necessarily because they have windsucker conformation.

It is well known that breeding problems are frequently associated with mares. What is often forgotten, or at least ignored, is the fact that stallions contribute 50 percent to a mating situation and problems can be encountered. Normal anatomical relationships must be considered before abnormal ones are understood.

Sperm are produced in each of the two *testicles* and stored in the epididymis associated with each testis. These structures are normally located outside the body wall, within a skin pouch, called the *scrotum*. Because sperm cannot be produced at normal body temperatures, the testicles have this external location. It should also be mentioned that even the blood flowing to these gonads is cooled through a tortuous system of the testicular vein called the *pampinform plexus*. Warmth from the arterial blood is transferred to the cooler venous blood. The result: blood entering the testicle is cooler than that leaving the body, and blood entering the body is warmer than that leaving the testicle. This same heat transfer principle is used in the pasteurization of milk.

The *ductus* ("vas") *deferens* are ducts passing through the nearby inguinal canal into the body. The function of each of these tubes is to transport sperm from the area of storage, the *epididymis*, to the main duct, leaving the body, the *urethra* during ejaculation.

Fluids are added to the volume of the ejaculate during mating from accessory genital glands associated with the stallion's reproductive

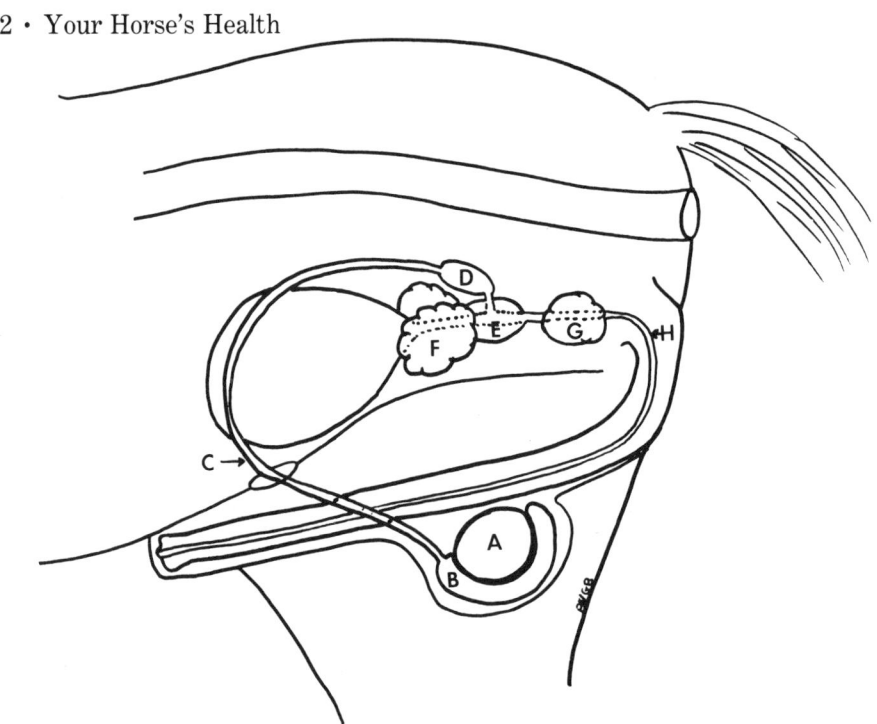

FIGURE 26. **Male Reproductive Tract, Side View: A–Testicle; B–Epididymus; C–Ductus Deferens; D–Ampulla; E–Prostate; F–Seminal Vesicle; G–Bulbourethral Gland; H–Urethra.**

tract. The *ampulla* of the ductus deferens is located surrounding each ductus deferens shortly before it opens into the urethra. The opening into the urethra is closely associated with two additional glands, the *prostate* which surrounds the urethra, and the *seminal vesicles*. Near the area where the urethra enters the external penis, the *bulbourethral glands* also add fluid. It is the cumulative production of the testes and the accessory sex glands that is ejaculated during breeding.

The urethra of the stallion connects the urinary bladder to the external environment. During its course inside the pelvic area both ductus deferens join it, as do ducts from most of the accessory genital glands. Once the urethra passes outside the body cavity it becomes surrounded by a great deal of vascular tissue and the entire structure becomes known as the *penis*. In cross section, the penis shows two separate areas of erectile, or vascular, tissue. The *corpus spongiosum penis* surrounds the urethra and the *corpus cavernosum penis* is located near it. The increased flow of blood into these areas and the decreased outflow result in the great increase in length and diameter of the penis observed during erection.

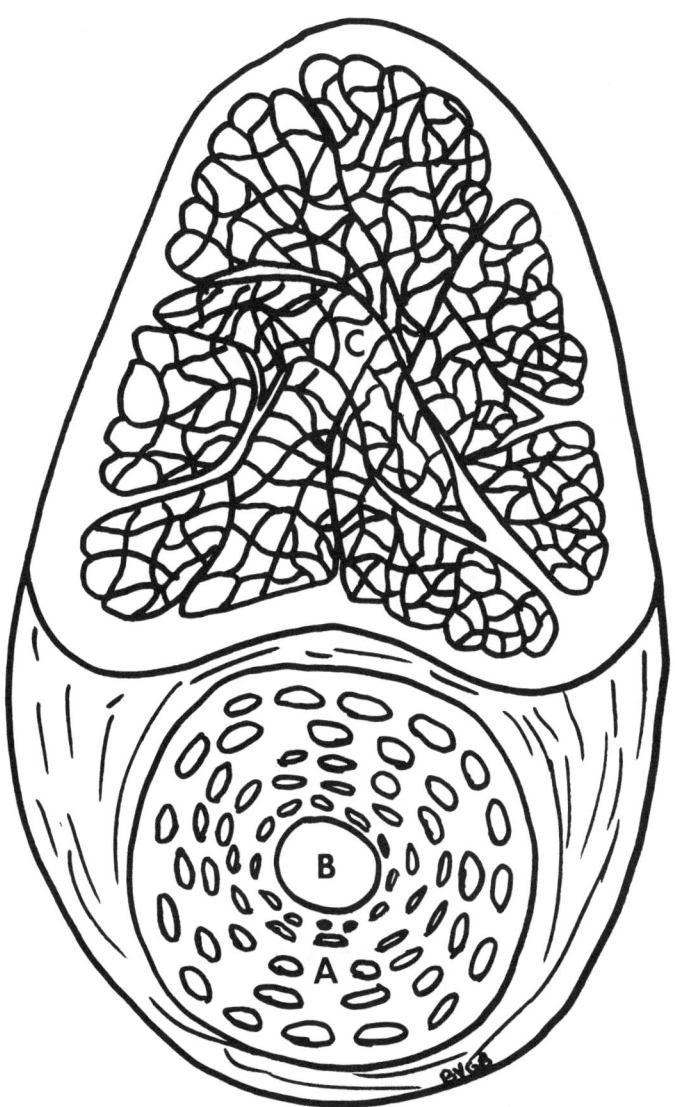

FIGURE 27. Cross Section of a Horse Penis: A–Corpus Spongiosum Penis; B–Urethra; C–Corpus Cavernosum Penis.

The area of penis observable during erection is normally kept within a skin pouch, the *prepuce*. The inner lining of the prepuce is extensive to accommodate the increased length during erection and thus is not seen in entirety unless full penile protrusion occurs. Slight protrusion, as during urination, leaves most of the prepucal lining covered. Grossly, the tip of the penis has a visable point, the *urethral process* where the urethra opens, and near it is a *diverticulum* or pocket. Smegma is an odoriferous substance normally produced within the prepuce, and on occasion this production may be excessive and appear as a prepucal swelling. In these males it is necessary to remove this buildup. Smegma may also accumulate within the uretheral diverticulum, dry out, and cause irritation during urination. The dried product is called a "bean," and must be removed to eliminate the problem.

The decision of which stallion will service a mare should be based on several factors, each considered carefully prior to the final selection. After all, if a foal is to be produced why settle for an individual inferior to or equal to the mare? Careful selection can upgrade an owner's investment.

The individual stallion is the usual reason many people give for

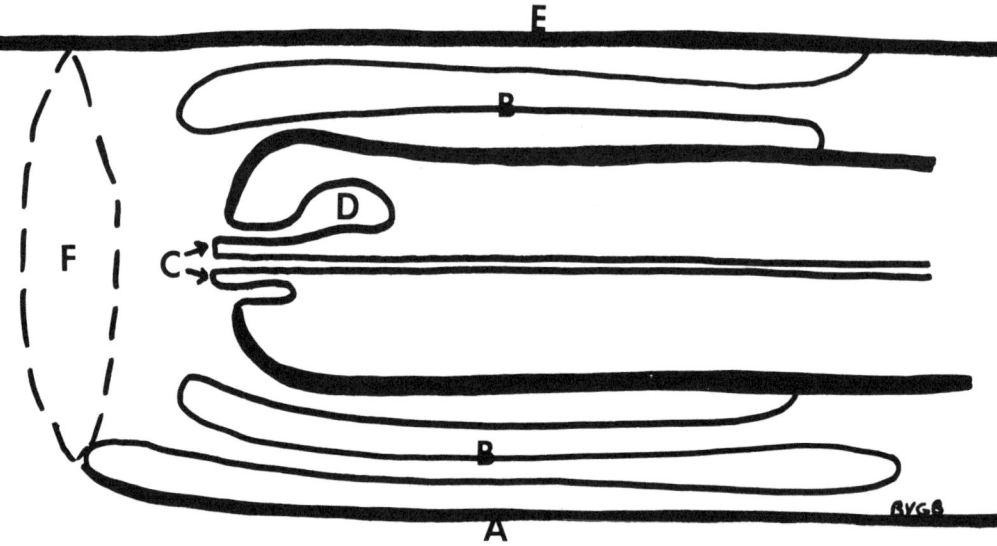

FIGURE 28. **Penis and Prepuce: A–Skin of the Prepuce; B–Lining of the Prepuce; C–Urethral Process; D–Diverticulum; E–Abdominal Wall; F–Opening of the Prepuce.**

selection. A horse may sell himself by his track or show record, or a pretty picture in some magazine. Show records, and to a lesser extent, track records, are poorly inheritable and selection by these factors alone does not produce consistant foal crops. Certain photographers have a real knack for bringing out the best in an average horse, and some super horses are not photogenic. Pictures can lie, visual inspection can't. An individual stallion's offspring will tell much more about the horse than any other single factor. By examining the foals and their records, the mare owner can obtain a much better picture of the stallion's reproductive capabilities. Do the offspring show strengths in areas where the mare has weaknesses—conformation, ability, behavior? Of course foals produced aren't always the best but by carefully evaluating the previous offspring of a stallion, guesswork can be minimized.

Pedigree selection is another method mare owners use to choose a stallion. As with the other methods, this one also has pros and cons. If the choice is made only because the stallion has a famous relative, big chances are being taken. Many pedigree types don't mix well, but careful selection using the principles of genetics can be of benefit in more rapidly upgrading a breeding program. Large genetic pools are available in most registries, and with the strong trend toward popularity of registered horses which also bring better prices, a horse breeder should give serious consideration to raising registered stock.

Cost factors should also be considered in stallion selection. The most obvious expense is the stud fee. A high fee does not guarantee an outstanding foal, but it does guarantee the foal must bring a high price just to break even. Hauling the mare to the stallion and mare care are additional expenses encountered. If the mare has a foal by her side a great deal of consideration should be given to the distance to be traveled. Veterinary bills for sick foals or for mares not in breeding condition can also add to the cost of the final product.

Stallion operations can be handled in several ways using pasture breeding, hand management, or artificial insemination. Many mare owners have preferences. Before selecting a stallion it would be to the mare owner's advantage to investigate the percentage of mares settled during the previous breeding seasons. Low percentages could indicate that a stallion was being used too heavily and it might also indicate that a mare owner could lose money and valuable time with an open mare.

The failure of a mare to produce a foal is not necessarily her fault. Many of the causes of conception failure can be traced to the male.

Live sperm are necessary for egg fertilization in the mare, and anything interfering with the production or transport of these tiny cells will affect the reproductive ability of the stallion. In individual males one or both testicles may not become located in the scrotum, remaining in or near the body cavity. Cryptorchids are rarely capable of siring offspring because the testicle temperature is too high for sperm production. These stallions can act like any stallion or often, because of higher testosterone production, the horse may be almost unmanageable. A more frequent occurence is the monorchid, an individual with one normal and one retained testicle. These stallions have one testicle capable of producing sperm so offspring are possible. There is a real problem to the horse population by allowing the monorchid to reproduce, however. The retention of testicles is an inheritable condition in horses, and stallions with one retained testicle usually produce colts which have one or both testicles retained, and fillies which in turn can produce colts with retained testicles. This certainly is undesirable from the behavior and reproductive standpoint, from the surgical standpoint for neutering such a male, and from the health standpoint because internal testicles are more prone to develop cancer and to be involved with other internal problems. It is best to carefully avoid breeding with stallions not having both testicles in the scrotum.

Infections of any part of the stallion genital tract can directly affect the quality and livability of sperm. This can involve inflammation of the testicles, epididymis, scrotum, or accessory sex glands. The causes of infection are quite variable. Infected mares can introduce the problem to a servicing stallion, it can be the result of an injury, or it can be part of a disease process infecting the entire animal. The outcome is also variable. The stallion may infect mares he services in some cases, he may show no after effects, or sperm production can be decreased even to the point of being nonexistant.

Another fairly common cause of fertility disturbances in the stallion is overuse. Sperm are constantly being produced and only a certain volume can be stored. Popular stallions which are used heavily, mating mainly by natural service, can exhaust the supply of mature sperm. Rest will restore the numbers to normal. The frequency with which a male can successfully mate within a given time period depends on the age of the animal and on the amount of service prior to the given time. Two- and three-year olds definitely cannot be used as heavily as aged stallions, usually one to three times weekly. Older animals can be used more heavily at ten or more services per week if a few days are given afterward to allow sperm production to catch up. Owners using stallions heavily during the breeding season risk the probability that many mares may not settle and that the stallion will then develop a poor breeding reputation.

With sound breeding practices, a breeder can get a mare in foal. At the time of conception a foal starts as the joining of two cells, one egg and one sperm, microscopic in size. From this union a foal will grow into an animal with millions of specialized cells. In the formation of this complex animal, several important things occur during the first three months of pregnancy.

Shortly after fertilization the cells start to divide and eventually get numerous enough to start forming the outer covering and the inner body "substance" from which internal structures will eventually form. The embryo at this time has no resemblance to the horse of the future, being just a tiny blob. A start of the brain and spinal cord are two of the first structures to form, and these are followed shortly by the start of the head and spinal column. Blood vessels appear and will be followed by the formation of the heart, soon to beat. Blood can now be pumped to the *placenta* ("afterbirth") for oxygen to nourish the rapidly multiplying cells. The eyes start forming, then the internal parts of the ears. Not long after the eyes and ears begin, the foal will have gills appearing, similiar to those of a fish. Gills, although looking remarkable in the fetus, last only a short time during the total growth period. As growth progresses from head end to tail end, the lungs will be next to start formation, although their formation won't be complete until almost the date of foaling. This long-term formation is one of the important reasons premature foals, or people, often die of lung problems. The lungs are not mature enough to handle the minute to minute business of breathing. The digestive system and the urinary system develop shortly after the start of the lung formation.

While the foal is carried by the mare it can not breathe, nor can it eat. Thus oxygen and nutrients must get to the foal through its bloodstream. The foal has special structures to carry this blood in and out of its body in the *umbilical cord*. These attach to the placenta, where the mother's blood gives up oxygen and nutrients to the foal's blood, and takes up its blood wastes. When the enriched blood gets back inside the foal it goes to the heart to get pumped to the body. In the adult horse, blood would normally have to go to the lungs and return to the heart before it could go to the body. In the foal the lungs aren't functioning, and the heart has two special holes in or near it to allow the blood to bypass the lungs. These holes will close within a few

78 · Your Horse's Health

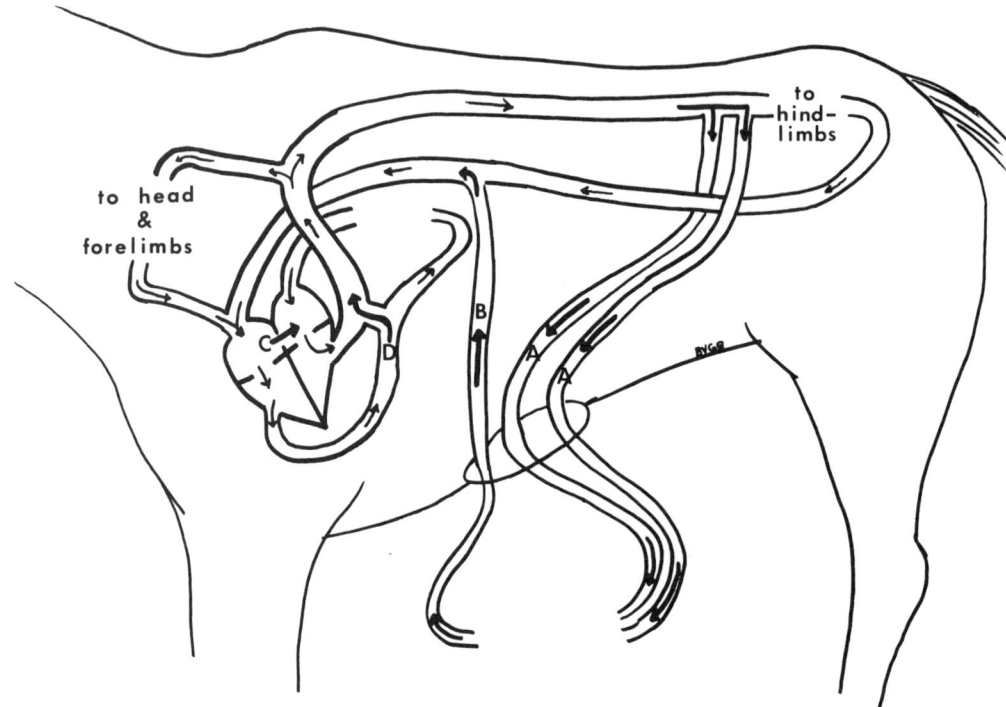

FIGURE 29. **Fetal Circulation: A–Umbilical Arteries; B–Umbilical Vein; C–Foramen Ovale; D–Ductus Arteriosus.**

days after birth. Blood flow in the unborn foal has two *umbilical arteries* carrying blood to the placenta, the *umbilical vein* returning blood to the foal, the normal major vessels of the foal's body, and two major blood shunts near the heart that bypass the lung, the *foramen ovale* and the *ductus arteriosus*.

The kidneys of the fetus function very early in development and their wastes go to the urinary bladder as they would in the adult. The urinary bladder of the adult is similiar to a water balloon, expandable and contractable. In the unborn foal the urinary bladder is a tube which goes out into the umbilical cord so that the dilute urine can be deposited in a pouch surrounding the fetus. At birth the rupture of this cavity containing the dilute urine is called "breaking of the water bag" and indicates a new foal will soon be born.

After a long wait the exciting day arrives and the mare gives birth to the little creature she has cared for so long. Parturition usually occurs at night for mares and so it is an event not often seen.

When a mare conceives, she provides the sheltered environment and nourishment needed by the unborn foal for 322 to 344 days. At the end of her pregnancy the mare goes into labor so that her body can position the foal for delivery into the world and actually push it out. The first stage of labor is outwardly seen as a slight increase in restlessness. Internally the cervix is starting to relax and dilate while the uterus is starting to contract. These contractions, called labor pains in women, occur approximately every fifteen minutes and last for fifteen to twenty seconds each. Restlessness increases as seen by the mare getting up and down frequently. In reality her muscular movements are helping position the foal in the birth canal. This first stage lasts from one-half to four hours.

Stage two of parturition in the mare starts when the "water bag" breaks. This is often subtle in horses and can easily be missed by the observer. Uterine contractions have become much more forceful and will now include straining of all body muscles. Delivery should occur in ten to thirty minutes from the start of this heavy straining, and if it doesn't get veterinary help immediately. After giving birth the mare may continue to lie for fifteen to twenty minutes, resting from her strenuous muscular activity.

Fetal membranes (placenta) are expelled during the third stage of birth. This occurs with mild contraction efforts from one-half to three hours after foaling. It is important to make sure that the entire placental sac was expelled because small pieces left can easily become infected or can cause a tissue reaction resulting in laminitis.

A newborn foal will develop responses to its environment shortly after birth. Its eyes can respond to light and its body to pain by ten minutes of age. The youngster will first successfully stand in fifteen minutes to three hours time (one hour is average). Unlike with a dog or cat, the foal's umbilical cord may not break for up to thirty minutes after birth, although eight minutes is a good average. It does finally break because of the foal's movements, not because of the dam chewing it.

The final stage of parturition in the mare is the involution of the uterus, the time the uterus takes to get back into its nonpregnant state. In a normal mare this phase lasts twenty-five to thirty days and should be an important consideration when deciding to rebreed. Most mares will come into heat four to fourteen days after foaling (nine days is average). For some breeders it is common practice to rebreed a mare during her foal heat. If we consider that the uterus is not yet in normal nonpregnant condition we can understand the following figures given by Dr. R. Zemjanis, a noted authority in reproduction at the University of Minnesota: mares bred in foal heat conceive 43 percent of the time, mares bred in the first heat after foal heat conceive 67 percent of the time. Of the 43 percent mares that do settle during a foal-heat breeding, there is a four-times higher rate of abortions and resorptions of the fetuses and a six-times higher rate of sick and diseased foals. Is breeding back early really worth the risk?

It is important to watch the foal after its birth, checking to be sure several things happen. Many horsemen will put iodine on the stump of the umbilical cord, the navel, shortly after birth to prevent infections from entering the foal's body at this vulnerable spot. Within a few hours the little horse should have a bowel movement, passing a dark sticky substance. If this substance isn't passed by the foal or if the observer doesn't have time to watch for its passage, an enema should be given. For this purpose the disposable enemas available in drug stores, for human use, work very well. Making sure the foal nurses soon after it stands is also an important observation to be made. Any newborn animal will go downhill rapidly if not allowed to nurse.

9
Nature's Telephone System (The Nervous System)

Communication between various parts of the horse's body is extremely important for coordination. One front limb must know what the other is doing and what the hind limbs are doing. If the eye sees a jump, the message must reach the feet as well. The nervous system functions as the switchboard of an internal "telephone system."

Within the mammal the nervous system is generally divided into two parts—the *Central Nervous System*, (CNS, the *brain* and *spinal cord*) and the *Peripheral Nervous System*, (PNS, the nerves which connect the CNS with muscles and viscera). Nerves of the PNS serve only as telephone wires, carrying messages to the CNS from muscles or visera (an afferent nerve), or from the CNS to a body part (an efferent nerve). Another term, *Autonomic Nervous System* (ANS), applies only to efferent nerves of the PNS going to viscera.

The switchboard portion of the nervous system is located within the skull and vertebral column. It is because of the importance of the brain and spinal cord that they are so well protected by bone. The brain has three regions, each unique in shape and function. The *cerebrum* is the largest area and is somewhat globular in shape. It is divided into right and left hemispheres by a deep *longitudinal fissure*. The size of this portion of the brain has evolved from almost nonexistant in primitive mammals to extremely well developed in the human. In fact, scientists have tried to equate the size of this region with the intelligence of

82 · Your Horse's Health

various animals. A characteristic of the cerebrum is the presence of many *gyri* "ridges" and *sulci* "folds" and their numbers have also been used to try to explain intelligence.

All sensory information comes into the cerebrum, where it is interpreted and coordinated to formulate a reaction. The smell and shape of a carrot are received in the visual and olfactory areas. Memory links the two with a pleasurable taste, so messages are sent to the muscle-control centers of another portion of the brain, the *cerebellum*, to eat the carrot.

Located behind the cerebrum, the cerebellum is cauliflower-like in appearance. Coordination of muscle movements occurs here, so that a limb moves smoothly forward and stops at the appropriate moment. In a few rare individuals this brain section does not grow normally and movements are obviously affected. As the animal tries to drink water, first the head is thrust deeply in, then pulled too far out, then trust not quite so deeply in, then pulled not quite as far out. This sequence repeats itself until the mouth reaches the position desired.

The *medulla oblongata* is the third and most basic portion of the brain. Located behind and below the other two areas, the medulla oblongata is required to function for life. Within it are areas to stimulate respiration and heart function. In addition, pathways to higher centers traverse here. Even in the most primitive of animals,

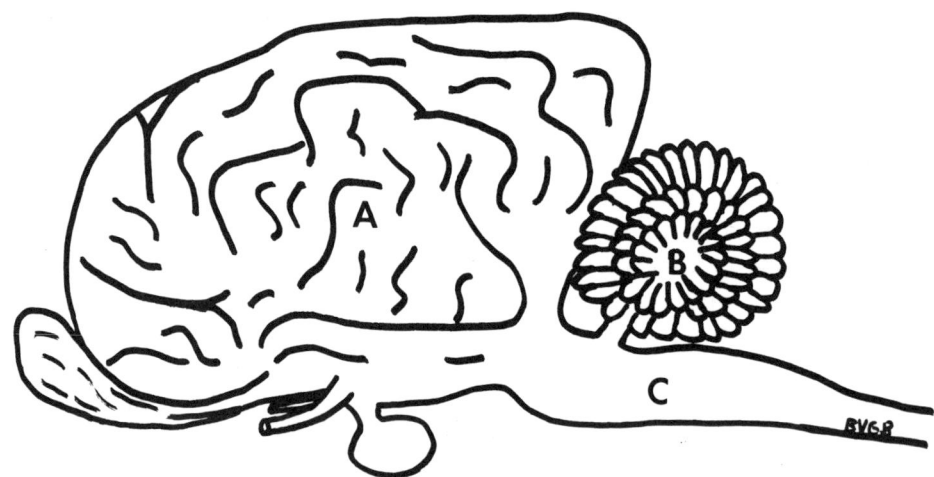

FIGURE 30. **The Brain: A–Cerebrum; B–Cerebellum; C–Medulla Oblongata.**

this area is present, if there is a nervous system, with the cerebrum and cerebellum added later in the evolutionary scale.

Although the spinal cord is basically a cable carrying messages to and from the various body parts, it does have the ability to help certain body parts react to emergency situations. For example, in the patellar reflex, a tap below the knee sends a message to the spinal cord which immediately directs the muscles of the thigh to kick the foot forward. The message doesn't have to take the longer route to the brain and back.

The brain is often called the "think center," gathering information in from all parts of the biologic machine and then evaluating this information to form a plan of attack. Scientists, however, are slow to gather unbiased information that animals can think—plan for the future. We can all cite instances when a horse "had to have reasoned" something out, but in forming that conclusion we usually have to assume some other particular human emotion or behavior is present.

To skirt the issue of thinking another question asks, "How smart is the horse as compared to other animals?" Depending upon which author you read, the list can start with anything from the elephant, to the dolphin, to the pig. The horse has been listed both near the top and bottom, just as other species have. All this confusion goes back to a few basic facts about intelligence and animals.

For humans, there are several different kinds of intelligence tests, but the simple fact remains that "intelligence" has never been satisfactorily defined, much less measured. The early environment of a child can greatly alter later results. So prior training and handling can alter the responses made by the horse. To measure intelligence we should not be measuring the ability of an animal to learn to do tricks.

Even if we could define intelligence quotient (I.Q.), how can we measure it in an unbiased manner? Human tests often involve visual discrimination, either in the form of words or pictures. Obviously, blind people will score low on these and thus would be classified "stupid." Individuals with auditory handicaps would probably fail vocal I.Q. tests. The problem is worse for animals, because in addition to obvious medical problems, results can be influenced by motivation. The desire for high scores may motivate an owner, but it is irrelevant to the horse. Motivational factors are highly variable, ranging from praise, to food, to punishment.

Add an additional complication—species variations. Individual equine variables are difficult enough, but now we want to compare the horse to other animals. Design of an I.Q. test becomes essentially impossible because of the great range of physical and behavioral differences. If the measure depended upon the positive response of a nose pushing a lever, the elephant would outrank the horse, which would outrank the cat. The reverse order of intelligence would be concluded if the positive response was a foot pushing a lever.

After all is said and done, there still is no quantitative way to define or measure intelligence, and the horse remains as smart as you want it to be.

Index

Abdomen, 55, 63, 65
Abortions, 79
Accessory genital glands, 71–72
Accessory sex glands, infection of, 76
Acetabulum, 34, 39
Adductor muscles, 32
Afterbirth, 77
Alveolus, 48
Ampulla, 72
ANS, 81
Anus, 55, 71
Aorta, 48, 51, 61
Aortic valve, 51
Arm, 15
Arteries: aorta, 48, 51, 61; cranial mesenteric, 56; coronary, 51; pulmonary, 51; renal, 61; umbilical, 78
Ascarids, 56
Atlas, 44
Atrioventricular valve: left, 51; right, 50
Atrium: left, 51; right, 50
Auricle, 50
Autonomic nervous system, 81
A–V valve: left, 51; right, 50
Axis, 44
Azoturia, 63–64

Baby teeth, 53
Bean, 74
Birth canal, 67, 79
Blood spavin, 41
Bloodworms, 55
Body of the uterus, 65, 66
Bog spavin, 41–42
Bone chips, 17

Bone fractures, 17
Bones: atlas, 44; axis, 44; calcanean tarsal bone, 36; cannon bone, 17, 24, 36, 39, 42; carpal bones, 17; cervical vertebrae, 44; coffin bone, 17, 19, 21, 28. 36; distal phalanx, 17, 19, 36; distal sesamoid bone, 19, 29; femur, 34, 35, 37, 39; fibula, 36; fibular tarsal bone, 36; humerus, 15, 17, 24, 25; ilium, 32; ischium, 32; long pastern bone, 17, 19, 25, 36; lumbar vertebrae, 44; metacarpal bones, 17, 24; metatarsal bones, 36; middle phalanax, 17, 19, 36; navicular bone, 19, 29, 39; patella, 34, 35, 41; pelvis, 32, 33, 34, 37, 39, 45, 63, 67; proximal phalanx, 17, 19, 36; proximal phalanx, 17, 19, 36; proximal sesamoid bones, 17, 36; pubis, 32; radius, 17, 24; ribs, 25, 44, 45, 46, 60; sacral vertebrae, 45; sacrum, 45; scapula, 15, 23, 24, 25, 26; short pastern bone, 17, 19, 25, 36; shoulder blade, 15, 25; splint bones, 17, 36; sternum, 45; thigh bone, 34; thoracic vertebrae, 44; tibia, 34, 35, 36, 37, 39; toe bone, 17; ulna, 17, 24; vertebral column, 44–45, 60, 77
Bone spavin, 42
Bot flies, 56
Bowman's capsule, 61, 62
Brain, 51, 60, 77, 81–83
Breaking of the water bag, 78, 79
Breeding cycles, 68
Bulhourethral glands, 72
Bursa, 43

Butazolidin, 30–31

Calcanean tarsal bone, 36
Cancer, 76
Cannon bone, 17, 24, 36, 39, 42
Cap, 53
Capillary, 51
Capped hock, 43
Carpal bones, 17
Carpus, 17
Caslick's operation, 71
Caudal vena cava, 49, 50, 63
Cecum, 55
Central incisor teeth, 53
Central nervous system, 81
Central tendon, 49
Cerebellum, 82, 83
Cerebrum, 81–82, 83
Cervical vertebrae, 44; atlas, 44; axis, 44
Cervix, 66, 79
Chest, 25, 44, 45, 48, 54
CNS, 81
Coffin bone, 17, 19, 21, 28, 36
Coffin joint, 19, 29, 36
Colic, 55, 56, 57–59
Collateral ligaments, 37
Colon, 55
Columns: major, 21, 28, 29; minor, 21, 28, 29
Common digital extensor muscle, 19, 28
Conformation, 21–28, 30, 37–41, 42, 43, 67, 69, 71, 75
Contracted tendons, 19
Coronary arteries, 51
Coronary band, 19, 28
Corner incisor teeth, 53
Corpus cavernosum penis, 72
Corpus spongiosum penis, 72
Cortex, 60, 61
Cranial mesenteric artery, 56
Cranial vena cava, 50
Croup, point of the, 32
Cruciate ligaments, 37
Crus, 36
Crus muscles, 48
Cryptorchid, 76
Curb, 42–43
Cuts, 19

Deciduous teeth, 53–54
Deep digital flexor muscle, 19, 25, 28, 29, 30

Diaphragm, 48, 49, 54
Diarrhea, 56
Distal phalanx, 17, 19, 36
Distal sesamoid bone, 19, 29
Diverticulum, 74
Ductus arteriosus, 78
Ductus deferens, 71, 72

Ear, 77
Egg, 65, 68, 69, 76, 77
Elbow, 17, 24, 25, 26
Elbows, out at the, 25
Embryo, 77
Epididymis, 71; infection of, 76
Epiglottis, 47, 52
Esophagus, 48, 54
Erectile tissue, 72
Estrous cycle, 67, 68, 70
Estrous period, 65
Eye, 77

Fallopian tube, 65
Fat horses, 70
Femur, 34, 35, 37, 39
Fetal membranes, 79
Fetal resorptions, 79
Fetlock, 17, 24, 25, 39
Fetus, 77, 78
Fibula, 36
Fibular tarsal bone, 36
Foal heat, 79, 80
Food tube, 54
Foot, 20, 24, 25, 26, 28, 39, 84
Foramen ovale, 78
Forearm, 17, 19
Founder, 19, 21, 28–29, 64
Frog, 20
Front limb, 15–31, 37, 41

Gaskin, 36
Gasterophilus species, 56
Gastrocnemius muscle, 36
Gills, 77
Glomerulus, 61
Gluteal muscles, 32
Grass founder, 28
Gyri, 82

Hard palate, 54
Head of the femur, 34
Heart, 50–51, 60, 77, 78
Heart attack, 51

Heart murmur, 51
Heart valves: aortic, 51; left atrioventricular, 51; pulmonary, 51; right atrioventricular, 50
Heat cycle, 67, 68
Heat period, 65, 67, 69, 70, 78, 79
Hind limb, 29, 32–43, 68
Hip, 32, 34, 39
Hock, 36, 39, 41, 42
Hoof, 19, 36
Hoof wall, 19, 20, 28
Hormones, 70
Human error, 70
Humerus, 15, 17, 24, 25

Ilium, 32
Incisor teeth, 53, 54
Infection of: accessory sex glands, 76; epididymis, 76; scrotum, 76; testicles, 76; uterus, 70; vagina, 70
Infertility, 76
Infundibulum, 65
Intelligence, 81, 82, 83–84
Intermediate incisor teeth, 53
Intestine: large, 55, 56; small, 54–55, 56
IQ, 83, 84
Ischiatic tuberosity, 32
Ischium, 32

Joint capsule, 41

Kidney, 60–62, 63, 78
Knee, 17, 19, 24, 25, 83
Kneecap, 34, 35, 41

Labor, 79
Laminitis, 28–29, 79
Large intestine, 55, 56
Larynx, 47
Lateral cartilages, 19
Left atrioventricular valve, 51
Left atrium, 51
Left A–V valve, 51
Left ventricle, 51
Leg, 36
Lips, 53
Ligaments, 24, 25, 26, 30, 31, 34, 35, 37, 41, 42, 43, 44
Liver, 55
Locked stifle, 41
Loin, 45, 63
Longitudinal fissure, 82

Long pastern bone, 17, 19, 25, 36
Lumbar vertebrae, 45
Lungs, 47, 48, 49, 51, 54, 60, 77, 78
Lymph, 51, 52
Lymph nodes, 52

Major columns, 21, 28, 29
Medial saphenous vein, 41
Medulla, 60, 61
Medulla oblongata, 82–83
Menisci, 37
Metacarpal bones, 17, 24
Metatarsal bones, 36
Middle phalanx, 17, 19, 36
Minor columns, 21, 28, 29
Monday morning disease, 63
Monoestrous breeding cycle, 68
Monorchid, 76
Mouth, 53, 54, 56
Muscles: adductor, 32; common digital extensor, 19, 28; crus, 48; deep digital flexor, 19, 25, 28, 29, 30; gastrocnemius, 36; gluteal, 32; muscular skirt, 48; superficial digital flexor, 19, 25;
Muscular skirt, 48

Navel, 80
Navicular bone, 19, 29, 30
Navicular disease, 19, 29–30
Nephron, 61, 62
Nose, 47, 54, 84

Obturator foramen, 32
Out at the elbows, 25
Ovarian cysts, 69, 70
Ovarian tumors, 69, 70
Ovary, 65, 69, 70
Overeating disease, 28
Oviduct, 65
Ovulation fossa, 65

Pampinform plexus, 71
Pancreas, 55
Parascaris equorum, 56
Parasites, 55–56
Partial impaction colic, 58
Pastern, 25, 30
Pastern joint, 17, 36
Patella, 34, 35, 41
Pelvic limb, 32–43
Pelvis, 32, 33, 34, 37, 39, 45, 63, 67
Penis, 72, 74
Periosteum, 19, 20, 21, 28

Peripheral nervous system, 81
Permanent teeth, 53–54
Phrenic nerve, 49
Pinworm, 56
Placenta, 77, 78, 79
Plantar ligament, 42
Pleura, 48
Pleurisy, 48
PNS, 81
Point of the: croup, 32; hip, 32; hock, 36, 42, 43; shoulder, 15, 17
Polyestrus, 68
Post-parturient laminitis, 28–29
Prepuce, 74
Primary bronchus, 48
Prostate, 72
Proximal phalanx, 17, 19, 36
Proximal sesamoid bones, 17, 36
Pubis, 32
Pulmonary: arteries, 51; valve, 51; veins, 51

Qxyuris equi, 56

Radius, 17, 24
Rectum, 55
Renal: arteries, 61; capsule, 60; pelvis, 61, 62; sinus, 61
Retention of testicles, 76
Ribs, 25, 44, 45, 46, 60
Right atrioventricular valve, 50
Right atrium, 50
Right A–V valve, 50
Right ventricle, 50, 51
Road founder, 28
Roaring, 47
Roundworms, 56

Sacral vertebrae, 45
Sacroiliac joint, 45
Sacrum, 45
Salpinx, 65
Scapula, 15, 23, 24, 25, 26
Scrotum, 71, 76; infection of, 76
Seminal vesicles, 72
Short pastern bone, 17, 19, 25, 36
Shoulder blade, 15, 23
Shoulder joint, 15, 23, 25
Sidebones, 19
Skin, 19, 20
Small intestine, 54–55, 56
Smegma, 74

Soft palate, 47, 54
Sole, 20, 28
Sore kidneys, 63
Sperm, 65, 66, 70, 71, 76, 77
Spinal cord, 44, 45, 77, 81, 83
Spine of the scapula, 15, 23
Spinous process, 44
Splint bones, 17, 36
Sternum, 45
Stifle, 23, 32, 34, 35, 37, 39, 41
Stomach, 54, 56
Strongyles, 55, 56
Strongyloides, 56
Strongylus vulgaris, 55, 58
Sulci, 82
Superficial digital flexor muscle, 19, 25
Sweeney, 15

Tapeworm, 56
Tarsal: bones, 36; joint, 36
Tarsus, 42
Teeth, 53, 54
Tendons, 24, 25, 34, 43
Testicle, 71, 76; infection of, 76
Testicular vein, 71
Testis, 71, 72
Testosterone, 76
Thigh bone, 34
Thoracic limb, 15–31, 37
Thoracic vertebrae, 44
Thorax, 48, 49, 54
Tibia, 34, 35, 36, 37, 39
Tied-up, 63
Toe bone, 17
Trachea, 47, 48, 54
Transitory polyoestrus, 68
Transverse processes, 44, 45
True polyoestrus, 68
Tuber coxae, 32
Tunica intima, 55, 56
Twisted intestines, 58, 59

Ulna 17, 24
Umbilical: arteries, 78; cord, 77, 78, 79, 80; vein, 78
Ureter, 62, 63
Urethra, 71, 72, 74
Urethral process, 74
Urinary bladder, 63, 72, 78
Urine, 62, 63, 71, 78
Uterine: horns, 65; tube, 65
Uterus, 65, 66, 71, 79; body of, 65, 66; infections of, 70

Vagina, 66, 67; infections of, 70
Vas deferens, 71
Veins: caudal vena cava, 49, 50, 63; cranial vena cava, 50; medial saphenous, 41; pampinform plexus, 71; pulmonary, 51; testicular, 71; umbilical, 78;
Ventricle: left, 51; right, 50, 51
Vertebral: column, 44–45, 60, 77; foramen, 44

Vestibule, 66, 67, 71
Vocal: cords, 47; folds, 47
Voice box, 47
Vulva, 67, 68, 71

Water founder, 28
Windpipe, 47, 54
Windsucker conformation, 71
Worming, 56–57

Vagina, 66, 67; infections of, 70
Vas deferens, 71
Veins: caudal vena cava, 49, 50, 63; cranial vena cava, 50; medial saphenous, 41; pampinform plexus, 71; pulmonary, 51; testicular, 71; umbilical, 78;
Ventricle: left, 51; right, 50, 51
Vertebral: column, 44–45, 60, 77; foramen, 44

Vestibule, 66, 67, 71
Vocal: cords, 47; folds, 47
Voice box, 47
Vulva, 67, 68, 71

Water founder, 28
Windpipe, 47, 54
Windsucker conformation, 71
Worming, 56–57